ADHD Rating Scale–IV
Checklists, Norms, and Clinical Interpretation

George J. DuPaul
Thomas J. Power
Arthur D. Anastopoulos
Robert Reid

THE GUILFORD PRESS
New York   London

D1262750

Published by The Guilford Press
A Division of Guilford Publications, Inc.
72 Spring Street, New York, NY 10012
http://www.guilford.com

Printed in the United States of America

This book is printed on acid-free paper.

Last digit is print number: 9 8 7 6 5 4 3 2

ISBN 1-57230-423-5

Preface

Attention-Deficit/Hyperactivity Disorder (ADHD) is one of the most common behavior disorders of childhood. Mental health and school practitioners are increasingly faced with the challenge of assessing children and adolescents who might have ADHD. After the publication of the *Diagnostic and Statistical Manual of Mental Disorders,* fourth edition (DSM-IV; American Psychiatric Association, 1994), we set out to create a brief questionnaire that would allow clinicians to quickly determine the frequency of ADHD symptoms. This manual presents the results of our efforts over the past 3 years. We believe that clinicians will find the ADHD Rating Scale–IV to be useful for a variety of activities, including screening, assessment, and the evaluation of treatment outcome.

It is important to note that this questionnaire represents a significant revision over the previously published ADHD Rating Scale (DuPaul, 1991). First, the items have been updated to reflect DSM-IV criteria. Second, the item responses have been altered slightly to reflect the frequency of behavior (i.e., responses range from "never or rarely" to "very often"). Third, we have collected extensive data on a normative sample that is representative of the U.S. population with respect to region, ethnic, and socioeconomic background. Finally, we present comprehensive data regarding the clinical utility of this scale for screening, diagnosis, and treatment evaluation purposes.

Of course, a project of this magnitude could not be completed without the support and assistance of many individuals. First, the investigation of the psychometric properties of the ADHD Rating Scale–IV was supported, in part, by a faculty research grant awarded to George DuPaul by Lehigh University. In addition, the efforts of our coinvestigators, Martin Ikeda and Kara McGoey, were integral to the completion of this project, particularly with respect to gathering reliability and validity data. We also greatly appreciate the assistance of the following individuals in obtaining normative, reliability, and validity data: John Baily, Michelle Beck, Al Bird, Michael Booher, Carol Caplan, Allison Costabile, Suzanne Cote, Ralph Daubert, Betty Donahue, Joanna Gabris, Harlene Galen, Vincent Glaub, Nina Hoover, Charlene Jennings, John Lestino, Daniel Martin, Michelle Nebrig, Mary Beth Noll, Nick Novak, Joe Olmi, Daniel Reschly,

Cynthia Riccio, Maura Roberts, Diana Rogers-Adkinson, Vincent Rutland, Scott Streck-enbein, James Stumme, and Emily Wien.

Given the increasing segment of the U.S. population for whom Spanish is the primary language, we enlisted the help of Amelia Lopez and Romilia Ramirez to translate the Home Version of the rating scale into Spanish. We are grateful to them for this effort. Finally, we appreciate the willingness of the thousands of parents and teachers who completed the ADHD Rating Scale–IV as part of our development of this scale.

Contents

CHAPTER 1

Introduction to the ADHD Rating Scales

Attention-Deficit/Hyperactivity Disorder (ADHD) is a diagnostic category used to describe individuals who display developmentally inappropriate levels of inattention, impulsivity, and/or motor activity (American Psychiatric Association, 1994). Approximately 1–5% of school-age children in the United States have ADHD, and these children are at high risk for scholastic underachievement, conduct problems, and problematic social relationships (Barkley, 1998; Hinshaw, 1994). Given the prevalence, chronicity, and myriad difficulties associated with this disorder, it is important for clinicians to use psychometrically sound instruments when evaluating children and adolescents suspected of having ADHD.

Purpose of the Manual

The purpose of this manual is to describe two behavior questionnaires (the ADHD Rating Scale–IV: Home Version and the ADHD Rating Scale–IV: School Version) that are based on the diagnostic criteria for ADHD as described in the fourth edition of the *Diagnostic and Statistical Manual of Mental Disorders* (DSM-IV; American Psychiatric Association, 1994). Information is presented about the development and standardization of these scales, collection of normative data, factor structure, psychometric properties (i.e., reliability and validity), as well as the interpretive uses of these scales in clinical and school settings.

Background and Description of the ADHD Rating Scale–IV

Over the past two decades, the diagnostic criteria for ADHD have undergone several changes that have significantly impacted the clinical assessment of this disorder. Consistent with recently espoused theoretical views of this disorder (e.g., Barkley,

1997), factor analyses of teacher ratings of ADHD symptoms according to the criteria of the third edition of the *Diagnostic and Statistical Manual of Mental Disorders* (DSM-III-R; American Psychiatric Association, 1987) have consistently revealed two separate factors of Inattention and Hyperactivity–Impulsivity (e.g., Bauermeister et al., 1995; DuPaul, 1991). Based, in part, on these findings, DSM-IV provides diagnostic criteria organized into two dimensions of Inattention and Hyperactivity–Impulsivity, each of which consists of nine symptoms.

An evaluation of ADHD typically includes diagnostic interviews with the child and his or her parents and teachers; behavior rating scales completed by parents and teachers, direct observations of school behavior, and clinic-based testing (Barkley, 1998; DuPaul & Stoner, 1994). Although many behavior questionnaires are available for use in such evaluations, very few of the currently available instruments specifically include items directly adapted from the DSM-IV criteria for ADHD. Thus, our purpose in creating the ADHD Rating Scale–IV was to provide clinicians with a method to obtain parent and teacher ratings regarding the frequency of each of the symptoms of ADHD based on DSM-IV criteria.

Eighteen scale items were written to reflect DSM-IV criteria as closely as possible while maintaining brevity. The primary change made to each symptom was to omit the word "often" from the symptomatic description because respondents are asked to indicate the frequency of each symptom on a 4-point Likert scale ("never or rarely," "sometimes," "often," or "very often"). Inattention symptoms comprise the odd-numbered items, and Hyperactive–Impulsive symptoms are represented by the even-numbered items. Alternating symptomatic items in this manner was an attempt to reduce response bias. Parents are asked to make a determination of symptomatic frequency that best describes the child's home behavior over the previous 6 months (in accordance with DSM-IV guidelines), and teachers rate the frequency that best describes the child's school behavior over the previous 6 months or since the beginning of the school year. English and Spanish versions of the ADHD Rating Scale–IV: Home Version are presented in the Appendix, as is the School Version of the ADHD Rating Scale–IV (English only).

Administration and Scoring

Both versions of the ADHD Rating Scale–IV are designed to be completed independently by a child's parent or teacher. The respondent is instructed to provide demographic information (i.e., name of child, age, grade, and name of respondent) and to circle the number for each item that best describes the child's home (or school) behavior over the previous 6 months (or since the beginning of the school year if the teacher has known the child for less than 6 months). If the respondent skips any item, he or she should be asked to provide a rating for this item. If the respondent indicates a lack of opportunity to observe the behavior and skips an item, then this item is not included in the scoring of the scale. If three or more items are omitted, the clinician should use extreme caution in interpreting the scale for screening, diagnostic, or treatment evaluation purposes.

The Home and School Versions of the ADHD Rating Scale–IV both consist of two subscales: Inattention (nine items) and Hyperactivity–Impulsivity (nine items). These subscales are empirically derived (see Chapter 2) and conform to the two symptomatic dimensions described in the DSM-IV. Thus, three scores (Inattention, Hyperactivity–Impulsivity, and Total) are derived from each version. The Inattention subscale raw score is computed by summing the item scores for the odd-numbered items (Items 1, 3, 5, 7, 9, 11, 13, 15, and 17). The Hyperactivity–Impulsivity subscale raw score is computed by summing the item scores for the even-numbered items (Items 2, 4, 6, 8, 10, 12, 14, 16, and 18). The Total Scale raw score is obtained by adding the Inattention and Hyperactivity–Impulsivity subscale raw scores.

Raw scores are converted to percentile scores by using the appropriate scoring profile (presented in the Appendix) based on the child's gender and age. The raw score for a particular gender, age, and scale is circled in the body of the profile. The corresponding percentile score is displayed in the extreme right- and lefthand columns of the profile. Figure 1.1 displays a sample profile for scoring the ADHD Rating Scale–IV: Home Version for a 7-year-old boy. This boy's mother provided ratings resulting in the following raw scores and percentiles: Hyperactivity–Impulsivity = 17 (95th percentile), Inattention = 13 (91st percentile), and Total = 30 (92nd percentile). Note that when a raw score is associated with more than one percentile score (as was the case for this boy's Total score), the clinician should report the *lowest* of the possible percentile scores.

In Chapter 2, we describe the factor analyses used to derive the subscales of the ADHD Rating Scale–IV. Descriptions of the normative samples, as well as gender, age, and ethnic differences in Scale scores, are given in Chapter 3. The reliability and validity of both versions of the ADHD Rating Scale–IV are detailed in Chapter 4. Chapters 5 and 6 provide clinicians with guidelines for the interpretation and use of the scales for diagnostic and treatment evaluation purposes.

ADHD RATING SCALE–IV: HOME VERSION
SCORING SHEET FOR BOYS

Child's name:_ Glenn Brown _____   Date:_ June 9, 1998 _____   Age:_ 7 _

%ile	HI 5–7	HI 8–10	HI 11–13	HI 14–18	IA 5–7	IA 8–10	IA 11–13	IA 14–18	Total 5–7	Total 8–10	Total 11–13	Total 14–18	%ile
99+	26	25	25	19	24	26	27	25	43	49	51	41	99+
99	25	24	24	18	23	25	26	24	42	48	50	40	99
98	22	21	21	16	20	22	24	23	40	42	47	36	98
97	21	18	18	16	20	19	22	19	37	37	38	32	97
96	19	17	18	15	18	18	21	18	36	34	37	30	96
95	(17)	17	18	13	16	17	20	17	34	31	35	28	95
94	17	15	18	12	15	16	19	16	33	29	34	27	94
93	17	15	16	11	15	15	18	15	30	27	34	27	93
92	16	14	16	11	14	15	18	14	(30)	26	33	26	92
91	16	14	15	11	(13)	14	18	14	29	26	32	25	91
90	15	13	14	10	13	14	18	14	29	25	31	23	90
89	14	13	13	10	12	14	17	13	28	24	30	21	89
88	14	12	12	10	12	13	17	12	27	24	30	21	88
87	13	11	11	9	12	13	16	12	25	23	28	20	87
86	13	11	10	9	12	12	16	11	22	23	26	20	86
85	12	10	10	8	11	12	14	11	22	22	23	19	85
84	12	10	9	8	11	12	14	10	21	21	22	18	84
80	11	9	8	7	9	11	10	9	19	20	19	16	80
75	9	8	7	6	8	9	9	8	18	17	14	13	75
50	5	4	3	2	5	6	5	4	10	10	7	7	50
25	3	2	1	0	2	3	2	1	6	5	4	3	25
10	1	0	0	0	0	0	1	0	2	1	1	0	10
1	0	0	0	0	0	0	0	0	0	0	0	0	1

Note. HI, Hyperactivity–Impulsivity; IA, Inattention.

FIGURE 1.1. Sample scoring profile on the ADHD Rating Scale–IV: Home Version for a 7-year-old boy.

CHAPTER 2

Factor Analysis

As delineated in the previous chapter, the diagnostic criteria for ADHD have undergone several changes that were due, in part, to variant conceptualizations of the dimensions underlying this disorder. During the 1960s and 1970s, ADHD was viewed as consisting of a single dimension of hyperactivity and inattention (American Psychiatric Association, 1968). As empirical investigations began to highlight the importance of problems with inattention and impulsivity in this syndrome, a tripartite model was developed wherein children had to meet criteria in three separate dimensions: inattention, impulsivity, and hyperactivity (American Psychiatric Association, 1980). Because there was a dearth of empirical data supporting this tripartite model, the diagnostic criteria were temporarily reconceptualized in DSM-III-R as constituting a unitary dimension (American Psychiatric Association, 1987).

Because the Home and School Versions of the ADHD Rating Scale–IV are based on the DSM-IV criteria for this disorder, we were interested in whether factor analyses of these scales would conform to the bidimensional structure of the diagnostic criteria list. Factor analyses would, in part, provide information about the construct validity of the two versions of this scale. Determining the structure of the scales would also help us to develop item lists for potential subscales for clinical purposes.

In this chapter we review two different factor analyses that were conducted for both versions of the ADHD Rating Scale–IV. Exploratory factor analyses provided us with initial information about the structure of these scales. Subsequent confirmatory factor analyses provided more specific information about the adequacy of the structural model presumed to underlie the two versions of the scale.

Sample and Procedures: Factor Analyses of the Home Version

Participants

The sample used to conduct factor analyses of the Home Version of the ADHD Rating Scale–IV included 4,860 children and adolescents between the ages of 4 and 20 from 22 school districts across the United States. Complete ratings of ADHD symptoms were available for 4,666 participants (2,470 girls, 2,134 boys, and 62 unspecified). Participants ranged in age from 4 to 20 years ($M = 9.57$; $SD = 3.33$) and attended kindergarten through 12th grade ($M = 4.17$; $SD = 3.27$). Participants were predominantly Caucasian ($n = 3,999$; 85.7%) with additional subjects identified as African-American ($n = 318$; 6.8%), Latino ($n = 105$; 2.3%), Asian-American ($n = 99$; 2.1%), Native American ($n = 13$; 0.3%), other ($n = 61$; 1.3%), and unspecified ($n = 71$; 1.5%).

Of the 4,666 respondents, the vast majority were mothers ($n = 4,071$; 87.2%), with additional ratings completed by fathers ($n = 494$; 10.6%), guardians ($n = 39$; 0.8%), grandparents ($n = 36$; 0.8%), and unspecified ($n = 26$; 0.5%). A total of 4,131 (88.5%) of the respondents were female, 524 (11.2%) were male, and 11 (0.2%) were unspecified. The age of respondents ranged from 19 to 80 years old ($M = 36.93$; $SD = 6.05$). As was the case for child participants, most parent/guardian respondents were Caucasian ($n = 4,063$; 87.1%), with additional respondents identifying themselves as African-American ($n = 295$; 6.3%), Latino ($n = 100$; 2.1%), Asian-American ($n = 87$; 1.9%), Native American ($n = 26$; 0.6%), other ($n = 52$; 1.1%), and unspecified ($n = 43$; 0.9%). The socioeconomic status of families was coded using a modified version of the Hollingshead Index (Hollingshead, 1975) based on the highest-status occupation in the household as reported by respondents. Hollingshead Indices ranged from 10 to 90 (10 to 30 = 20.5%; 31 to 60 = 30.5%; 61 to 90 = 43.5%; missing = 5.5%) with a median of 60 ($M = 58.05$; $SD = 23.46$) indicative of middle class socioeconomic status.

Procedures

The factor analytic sample was recruited by distributing the ADHD Rating Scale–IV: Home Version and a letter inviting participation in the study to students in kindergarten through 12th grade in 22 school districts across the United States. The letter outlined the potential risks and benefits associated with participating in the study. Parental consent was assumed if parents returned completed ratings. School districts were selected to represent urban, suburban, and rural locales so that geographic locations were sampled in accordance with U.S. Census data. In suburban/rural locations ($n = 14$), parent rating packets were distributed to every student in all districts. In larger urban locales ($n = 8$), because it was not practically possible to distribute packets to every student in a district, schools at the elementary and secondary levels were selected by school district administrators to provide a cross-section of the community. Parent rating packets were then distributed by classroom teachers to all students at each selected school. Ratings were completed between October and May in either the 1994–1995 or 1995–1996 school year, with return rates ranging from 22 to 40% ($M = 30%$) across school districts.

Sample and Procedures: Factor Analyses of the School Version

Participants

The sample used to analyze the factor structure of the School Version of the ADHD Rating Scale–IV consisted of 4,130 children and adolescents between the ages of 4 to

19 from 31 school districts across the United States. Complete ratings of ADHD symptoms were available for 4,009 participants (2,054 boys, 1,934 girls, and 21 unspecified). Students ranged in age from 4 to 19 years (M = 10.3; SD = 3.5) and attended kindergarten through 12th grade (M = 4.8; SD = 3.5). Participants were predominantly Caucasian (n = 2,785; 69.5%), with additional subjects identified as African-American (n = 735; 18.3%), Latino (n = 229; 5.7%), Asian-American (n = 74; 1.8%), Native American (n = 4; 0.1%), other (n = 119; 3.0%), and unspecified (n = 63; 1.6%). Most participants attended general education (n = 3,612) versus special education (n = 336) classrooms. A total of 2,005 teachers (1,605 female, 371 male, and 29 unspecified) participated, most completing ratings on one boy and one girl in their classrooms. As was the case for child participants, most teachers were Caucasian (n = 1,817; 90.6%), with additional teachers identifying themselves as African-American (n = 113; 5.6%), Latino (n = 25; 1.2%), Asian-American (n = 5; 0.2%), Native American (n = 1; < 0.1%), other (n = 13; 0.6%), and unspecified (n = 31; 1.5%). There was a wide range in years of teaching experience (0 to 44 years; M = 14.6; SD = 9.24).

Procedures

The factor analytic sample was obtained by asking teachers in the 31 districts to complete an ADHD Rating Scale–IV in regard to the performance of two randomly selected students (one boy and one girl) from their classrooms. Parental consent to participate was not obtained because ratings were anonymous and confidential. Teachers were asked to rate the behavior of students located at differing points on their class roster (e.g., fifth girl and eighth boy). Teachers at the secondary level, who taught more than one class, were asked to rate two randomly selected students from a randomly selected class (e.g., third period). In districts in suburban/rural locations (n = 22), all teachers were asked to participate. In the larger urban districts (n = 9), schools at each level were selected to provide a cross-section of the community, and all teachers at selected schools were invited to participate. Ratings were completed between October and May in either the 1994–1995 or 1995–1996 school year, with estimated return rates ranging from 50 to 95% (M = 85%) across school districts.

Exploratory Factor Analyses

Factor analyses for the ADHD Rating Scale–IV: Home and School Versions utilized a three-step data analysis procedure for each scale analyzed. First, we used a traditional factor extraction approach (which treats data as interval level) using principal-axis factoring (PAF) and oblique rotation, which allows factors to correlate. Second, we computed a forced one-factor solution (i.e., a solution in which only one factor was allowed), which served as a baseline. Third, we computed an unforced solution that extracted and rotated all factors with eigenvalues greater than 1.0. This solution was compared with the baseline solution to determine whether it significantly increased the variance accounted for.

This three-step approach represents a departure from the manner in which ADHD rating scales have been analyzed in previous studies—namely, the use of principal-component analysis (PCA) with varimax rotation (Reid, 1995). The shortcomings of the latter approach have previously been noted (e.g., Taylor & Sandberg, 1984). PCA, although commonly used, is not true factor analysis; rather, it is intended to create uncorrelated linear combinations of observed variables that explain as much total sample variance as possible. In contrast, true factor analysis attempts to find a solution that maximizes variance between groups of related variables.

Varimax rotation is questionable for two reasons (Gorsuch, 1983). First, varimax implies that factors are orthogonal or conceptually unrelated; however, previous studies have reported high correlations between Hyperactivity and Inattention factor scores (e.g., McCarney, 1989); thus, its use for the ADHD Rating Scale–IV seemed questionable. Second, the varimax procedure mitigates against producing a general factor solution and may create several "splinter" factors that could be more parsimoniously combined. In scales with high internal consistency (which suggests the possibility of a general factor), data should be obliquely rotated (Gorsuch, 1983).

Home Version Results

Analysis was performed on a sample of 4,666 participants for whom complete data were available. PAF analysis resulted in a two-factor solution that accounted for 51.8% of variance. Table 2.1 shows the factor loadings and communalities for the one-factor and two-factor solutions. The forced one-factor solution accounted for 45% of variance. The subsequent unforced PAF analysis resulted in a two-factor solution. Eigenvalues for factors were 8.16 and 1.16. After factor rotation, Factor 1 (Hyperactivity–Impulsivity) accounted for 25% of explained variance, and Factor 2 (Inattention) accounted for 22%.

Table 2.2 shows the structure matrix for the two-factor solution. The structure matrix is equivalent to a matrix of correlation coefficients between the item and the underlying latent factor. Because we used oblique rotation, the pattern matrix and structure matrix differ. The two-factor model resulted in a significant increase in fit over the one-factor model ($\chi^2 = 178$; $df = 1$; $p < .01$). Even-numbered items (reflecting Hyperactivity-Impulsivity) loaded on Factor 1, and odd numbered items (reflecting Inattention) loaded on Factor 2. Items 3, 15, and 5 loaded on both Hyperactivity and Inattention factors. The correlation between factors was –.68, indicating that the factors are closely related.

School Version Results

Analysis was performed on a sample of 4,008 participants for whom complete data were available. Table 2.3 shows the factor loadings and communalities for the one-factor and unforced solutions. The forced one-factor solution accounted for 64.8% of variance. As Table 2.3 indicates, all item loadings were in the .7 to .8 range. The subsequent unforced PAF analysis resulted in a two-factor solution that accounted for 71.9% of variance. Eigenvalues (and percent of variance) explained for Factors 1 and 2, respectively, were

TABLE 2.1. Rotated Pattern Matrix for the ADHD Rating Scale–IV: Home Version

| | Forced one-factor solution | | Two-factor solution | | |
| | | | | Loadings | |
	Communality	Loadings	Communality	Factor 1	Factor 2
Item 10	.35835	.59987	.47794	.76775	.12008
Item 16	.50100	.70781	.57818	.75000	–.01508
Item 18	.49285	.70203	.56139	.72829	–.03022
Item 6	.42957	.65541	.50463	.71635	.00879
Item 12	.34804	.58995	.42422	.68179	.04588
Item 14	.35727	.59772	.41007	.63189	–.01232
Item 4	.42224	.64980	.46180	.62665	–.07430
Item 8	.44414	.66568	.47224	.60366	–.11480
Item 2	.43105	.65655	.45803	.59161	–.11680
Item 7	.47420	.68863	.61860	–.03691	–.81126
Item 11	.44460	.66678	.58334	–.04286	–.79239
Item 9	.48835	.69882	.60751	.00814	–.77385
Item 1	.35835	.59863	.48443	–.06770	–.74049
Item 17	.46853	.68449	.55517	.05519	–.70631
Item 13	.41961	.64777	.46755	.11642	–.59896
Item 3	.57586	.75886	.57653	.35642	–.46984
Item 15	.61303	.78296	.61165	.38528	–.46656
Item 5	.46566	.68239	.46347	.34952	–.39239

TABLE 2.2. Rotated Structure Matrix for the ADHD Rating Scale–IV: Home Version

	Factor 1	Factor 2		Factor 1	Factor 2
Item 16	.76030	–.52730	Item 7	.51714	–.78605
Item 18	.74893	–.52761	Item 9	.53664	–.77941
Item 6	.71035	–.48045	Item 11	.49831	–.76312
Item 10	.68574	–.40426	Item 17	.53758	–.74401
Item 8	.68206	–.52707	Item 15	.70392	–.72969
Item 4	.67739	–.50227	Item 3	.67731	–.71326
Item 2	.67138	–.52085	Item 1	.43802	–.69425
Item 12	.65046	–.41975	Item 13	.52548	–.67847
Item 14	.64030	–.44387	Item 5	.61751	–.63110

Note. Adapted from DuPaul, Anastopoulos, et al. (1998). Copyright 1998 by Plenum Publishing Corporation. Adapted by permission.

TABLE 2.3. Rotated Pattern Matrix for the ADHD Rating Scale–IV: School Version

| | Forced one-factor solution | | Two-factor solution | | |
	Communality	Loading	Communality	Factor 1	Factor 2
Item 14	.51395	.71690	.70173	.93235	.14384
Item 18	.67337	.82059	.82190	.92376	.02472
Item 16	.64720	.80449	.79978	.92227	.04051
Item 10	.59497	.77134	.69933	.82345	−.01812
Item 12	.56392	.75094	.65439	.78556	−.03285
Item 6	.54949	.74127	.61623	.72938	−.07655
Item 4	.65826	.81155	.70977	.72826	−.15270
Item 8	.63222	.79512	.66390	.66339	−.19818
Item 2	.67876	.82272	.68186	.56983	−.31917
Item 7	.60135	.77546	.78576	−.11140	−.96105
Item 9	.65078	.80671	.79478	−.03427	−.91522
Item 11	.60234	.77611	.73550	−.03509	−.88187
Item 17	.60135	.78963	.75199	−.01957	−.88079
Item 1	.58827	.76699	.69768	−.00052	−.83564
Item 3	.71569	.84599	.76067	.17971	−.73660
Item 13	.60568	.77825	.66263	.11365	−.73022
Item 15	.76944	.87718	.78440	.29200	−.65596
Item 5	.62186	.78858	.62628	.30040	−.55108

Note. From DuPaul et al. (1997). Copyright 1997 by the American Psychological Association. Reprinted by permission.

11.38 (63.2%) and 1.57 (8.7%). After factor rotation, each factor accounted for 33% of explained variance. The sum is less than the 71.9% total because factors were allowed to correlate and the loadings reflect only unique variance. The two-factor model resulted in a significant increase in fit over the one-factor model ($\chi^2 = 191$; $df = 1$; $p < .01$).

Table 2.4 shows the structure matrix for the two-factor solution. The pattern matrix approximates simple structure. Even-numbered items (reflecting Hyperactivity–Impulsivity) loaded on Factor 1, and odd-numbered items (reflecting Inattention) loaded on Factor 2. As was the case for the Home Version, the pattern matrix suggests two distinct factors, one representing Hyperactivity and one Inattention. However, in contrast to the parent rating data, loadings tended to be higher, and the Inattention factor was more distinct. Only items 2 and 5 dual-loaded on both factors; however, the values of loadings of the second factor were relatively low. The correlation between factors was −.70, indicating that the factors are closely related.

Some items (e.g., items 7, 9, 14, 18, and 16) exhibited extremely high loadings. Because of the fact that loadings of this magnitude make it difficult to distinguish an item from the underlying factor itself, and that a small number of items with extremely high

TABLE 2.4. Rotated Structure Matrix for the ADHD Rating Scale–IV: School Version

	Factor 1	Factor 2		Factor 1	Factor 2
Item 18	.90641	−.62358	Item 9	.60803	−.89117
Item 16	.89384	−.60674	Item 7	.56306	−.88287
Item 10	.83616	−.59601	Item 17	.59857	−.86706
Item 4	.83543	−.66379	Item 3	.69665	−.86272
Item 14	.83140	−.51048	Item 15	.75235	−.86089
Item 12	.80861	−.58415	Item 11	.58381	−.85725
Item 8	.80248	−.66375	Item 1	.58593	−.83527
Item 2	.79383	−.71908	Item 13	.62612	−.80999
Item 6	.78310	−.58843	Item 5	.68714	−.76190

loadings may distort factor structure, we ran additional exploratory analyses using the same procedures. In each subsequent analysis we excluded one of the items with a high loading. Exclusion of items did not result in any discernible change in the factor structure or great disparity in the loading of other items.

Confirmatory Factor Analyses

Factor extraction methods typically utilize a matrix of Pearson product–moment correlations; however, this method assumes that variables are at least interval-level data. For ordinal data, such as rating scales, it is better to utilize polychoric correlations (Joreskog & Sorbom, 1993). Moreover, if item distributions are similar, as is the case with these data in which all items have a positive skewed distribution, spurious factors may emerge as a result of similarities between item distributions. To address these problems, we used linear structural equation modeling (LISREL 8) to perform a confirmatory factor analysis (CFA), using polychoric correlations and an asymptotic covariance matrix, to test the results of the PAF solution. This allows for cross-validation of the results of the exploratory analysis in that we started with a priori models (i.e., a baseline one-factor model and the two-factor model suggested by DSM-IV) and then assessed how well the model fit observed data (as opposed to the exploratory approach, which created a model from observed data). It also avoids violation of the assumption of a normal distribution, because the weighted least-squares estimation method is considered an asymptotic distribution-free estimator (Raykov & Widaman, 1995).

We computed two models, a one-factor model in which all items were constrained to load on one factor, and a two-factor model in which odd-numbered items were constrained to load on an Inattention factor and even-numbered items were con-strained to load on a Hyperactivity–Impulsivity factor. We analyzed the goodness-of-fit of both models (i.e., the extent to which the models accurately reproduced the observed correlation matrices) through comparison of multiple goodness-of-fit indices.

We should note that the results of structural modeling analysis are not straightforward. Because there is no single generally accepted index of model fit (Bollen, 1990), and because very large sample sizes can affect fit indices (Marsh, Balla, & McDonald, 1988), the process is rather one of interpretation through analysis and comparison of multiple fit indices, than one of simply rejecting (or failing to reject) the null hypothesis based on a test statistic. In addition, we should caution that even if a given model can be said to fit the data, it is incorrect to assume that this is *the correct model* that best fits the data. The results of structural equation modeling do not allow for this inference. The most appropriate inference is that the model in question is *a possible model* that adequately represents observed data.

Home Version Results

Table 2.5 shows fit indices for the Home Version data. The root mean square error of approximation (RMSEA; which is a measure of discrepancy per degree of freedom; Joreskog & Sorbom, 1993) of both models is below the .05 value, thereby indicating good fit. Moreover, the test of RMSEA is 1.00 for both models, also suggesting a good fit. This is consistent with the observed values of the goodness-of-fit index (GFI) and the adjusted GFI (AGFI). These indices range from 0 (equals no fit) to 1.0 (equals perfect fit) with values at or above .90 indicative of adequate fit, which suggests that both models fit the data well. The Parsimony GFI (PGFI), which applies a correction for sample size, is also high for both models. These results suggest that both models adequately fit observed data. Other estimates of comparative fit—the normal fit index (NFI), parsimony NFI (PNFI), comparative fit index (CFI), incremental fit index (IFI), and relative fit index

TABLE 2.5. Goodness-of-Fit Indices for the ADHD Rating Scale–IV: Home Version for One-Factor and Two-Factor Models

Fit index	Index value	
	One-factor model	Two-factor model
Model $\chi^2(df)$	1,625 (135)	1,447 (134)
RMSEA	.049	.046
p value for test of close fit (RMSEA < .05)	1.00	1.00
GFI	.98	.98
AGFI	.97	.97
PGFI	.77	.77
NFI	.93	.94
PNFI	.82	.82
CFI	.94	.95
IFI	.94	.95
RFI	.93	.93

Note. RMSEA, root mean square error of approximation; GFI, goodness-of-fit index; AGFI, adjusted goodness-of-fit index; PGFI, parsimony adjusted goodness-of-fit index; NFI, normed fit index; PNFI, parsimony normed fit index; CFI, comparative fit index; IFI, incremental fit index; RFI, relative fit index.

(RFI)—which assess the extent to which the restricted model (i.e., the one-factor and two-factor) improves fit over a null model (which also ranges from 0 to 1, with values above .9 indicating good fit) suggest that there is little difference between models.

School Version Results

Table 2.6 shows fit indices for the School Version data. These results are quite similar to those of the Home Version data. The RMSEA of both models is near the 0.05 value, indicating close fit. In addition, the test of RMSEA is 1.00 for both models also indicating a good fit. This is consistent with the observed values of GFI and AGFI. The PGFI is also high for both models. Other estimates of comparative fit, the NFI, PNFI, CFI, IFI, and RFI, suggest that there is little difference between models.

Summary and Conclusions

The results of both exploratory and confirmatory factor analyses of the ADHD Rating Scale–IV indicate that either a one- or two-factor solution would best represent the structure of this scale. Because some results favored the two-factor solution, which conformed with the DSM-IV bidimensional diagnostic criteria, we decided to construct two subscales for each version of the ADHD Rating Scale–IV. Odd-numbered items can be totaled to derive an Inattention subscale score, and even-numbered items can be summed to obtain a Hyperactivity–Impulsivity subscale score. These two scale scores can then be used by clinicians to determine a child's normative status in respect to the two domains of DSM-IV symptoms of ADHD. Separate scale scores may also aid in determining the ADHD subtype for a specific child (see Chapters 3 and 5).

TABLE 2.6. Goodness-of-Fit Indices for the ADHD Rating Scale–IV: School Version for One-Factor and Two-Factor Models

	Index value	
Fit index	One-factor model	Two-factor model
Model $\chi^2(df)$	1,730 (135)	1,539 (134)
RMSEA	.054	.051
p-value for test of close fit (RMSEA < .05)	1.00	1.00
GFI	.99	.99
AGFI	.99	.99
PGFI	.78	.78
NFI	.98	.99
PNFI	.87	.86
CFI	.99	.99
IFI	.99	.99
RFI	.98	.98

CHAPTER 3

Standardization and Normative Data

The primary purpose of this chapter is to describe the process of obtaining normative data for the Home and School Versions of the ADHD Rating Scale–IV. Two nationally representative samples were used to derive normative data (as reported in DuPaul et al., 1997; DuPaul, Anastopoulos, et al., 1998). Differences in parent and teacher ratings as a function of age, gender, and ethnic group are also discussed. Finally, we present epidemiological data regarding the prevalence of ADHD subtypes in our normative samples.

Development of Normative Data: Samples and Procedures

ADHD Rating Scale–IV: Home Version

Participants

The normative sample consisted of 2,000 (1,043 girls, 930 boys, and 27 unspecified) randomly selected participants from the overall sample used for factor analyses (see Chapter 2). Participants ranged in age from 4 to 20 years ($M = 9.63$; $SD = 3.53$) and attended kindergarten through 12th grade ($M = 4.21$; $SD = 3.46$). As described in the following paragraphs, this sample was selected to approximate U.S. Census (1990) data distributions for ethnic group and region (see Table 3.1).

Parent/guardian respondents (1,753 female, 244 male, and 3 unspecified) ranged in age from 19 to 80 years ($M = 37.12$; $SD = 6.35$). Parent/guardians were predominantly Caucasian ($n = 1470$; 73.5%), with additional respondents identifying themselves as African-American ($n = 285$; 14.2%), Latino ($n = 93$; 4.7%), Asian-American ($n = 86$; 4.3%), Native American ($n = 14$; 0.7%), other ($n = 47$; 2.4%), or of unspecified ethnic background ($n = 5$; 0.3%). Most of the respondents were mothers ($n = 1,711$; 85.6%) with remaining ratings provided by fathers ($n = 226$; 11.3%), grandparents ($n = 23$; 1.2%), guardians ($n = 21$; 1.1%), and unspecified ($n = 19$; 1.0%). Families were living primarily in middle-class socioeconomic circumstances, with a median Hollingshead

TABLE 3.1. Percentage of Participants in Normative Sample by Region and Ethnic Group for the ADHD Rating Scale–IV: Home Version

	Percentage in sample	U.S. Census percentage[a]
Region		
Northeast	25.5	20.0
Midwest	25.2	24.0
South	28.0	34.0
West	21.3	21.0
Ethnic group		
White, non-Latino	70.2	74.8
African-American	15.9	11.9
Latino	5.3	9.5
Native American	0.7	0.7
Asian-American	5.0	3.1
Other	3.1	—

Note. From DuPaul, Anastopoulos, et al. (1998). Copyright 1998 by Plenum Publishing Corporation. Reprinted by permission.

[a]Percentages are from 1990 U.S. Census data.

Index of 60 (ranging from 10 to 90; 10 to 30 = 22.2%; 31 to 60 = 28.6%; 61 to 90 = 43.3%; missing = 5.9%; M = 56.16; SD = 24.52).

Measures

Parents and guardians were asked to complete a two-page packet. On the first page, parents provided information regarding their age, sex, relationship to the child, occupation, spouse's occupation, and ethnic group. Information also was provided about the child being rated, such as age, sex, grade, and ethnic group. The second page of the packet included the ADHD Rating Scale–IV: Home Version. Parents selected the single response for each item that best described the frequency of the specific behavior displayed by the target child over the past 6 months.

Procedures

Normative data were obtained by selecting a subsample of ratings from the factor analytic sample (see Chapter 2 for description of sampling procedures) so as to conform, as closely as possible, to U.S. Census data population proportions regarding region and ethnic group. Participants were randomly selected from the factor analytic sample in a stratified manner (i.e., random selection was constrained to conform with proportions of regional and ethnic distribution). Percentages of children by region and ethnic group are displayed in Table 3.1 relative to corresponding percentages in the 1990 U.S. Census. The resulting normative sample closely matches U.S. Census distributions for region, with the exception of the Southern part of the United States, which is somewhat underrepresented in the sample (i.e., 27.8% in the sample versus 34% in the Census). The Northeastern region is slightly overrepresented in the normative sample (i.e., 25.4% in the sample versus 20% in the Census). African-Americans (15.9% in the sample versus 12% in the Census) were slightly overrepresented in the normative group. Nevertheless, differences between sample proportions and U.S. Census data are minimal; thus, we consider the normative sample to be representative of the U.S. population.

ADHD Rating Scale–IV: School Version

Participants

The normative sample consisted of 2,000 (1,040 boys, 948 girls, and 12 unspecified) randomly selected participants from the factor analytic sample described in Chapter 2. As described in the following paragraphs, this sample was selected to approximate U.S. Census (1990) data distributions for ethnic group and region. Participants ranged in age from 4 to 19 years ($M = 10.6$; $SD = 3.6$) and attended kindergarten through 12th grade ($M = 5.1$; $SD = 3.5$). Most children attended general education ($n = 1,816$) versus special education ($n = 161$) classrooms. The racial distribution of the sample was 65.1% Caucasian ($n = 1,303$), 18.5% African-American ($n = 369$), 8.0% Latino ($n = 160$), 1.7% Asian-American ($n = 34$), 0.2% Native American ($n = 3$), and 5.2% other ($n = 104$), with an additional 27 participants (1.4%) of unspecified ethnic origin. Participants were identified as living in one of four regions of the United States, 34.0% ($n = 680$) from the South, 29.5% ($n = 590$) from the Midwest, 20% ($n = 400$) from the Northeast, and 16.5% ($n = 330$) from the West. A total of 1,001 teachers (793 female, 194 male, and 14 unspecified) completed ratings. Teachers were predominantly Caucasian ($n = 902$; 90.2%), with additional teachers identifying themselves as African-American ($n = 61$; 6.1%), Latino ($n = 13$; 1.3%), Asian-American ($n = 3$; 0.3%), Native American ($n = 1$; 0.1%), other ($n = 6$; 0.6%), or of unspecified ethnic background ($n = 15$; 1.5%).

Measures

Teachers for both samples were asked to provide information regarding their gender, ethnic group, and years of teaching experience as well as the type of classroom (general or special education) and the grade level they taught. Information about the child being rated, such as gender, ethnic group, and age was also provided. Teachers completed the ADHD Rating Scale–IV: School Version. Teachers selected the single response for each item that best described the frequency of the specific behavior displayed by the target child over the past 6 months (or since the beginning of the school year).

Procedures

Normative data were obtained by selecting a subsample of ratings from the factor analytic sample (see Chapter 2 for description of sampling procedures) so as to conform, as closely as possible, to U.S. Census data population proportions regarding region and ethnic group. Participants were randomly selected from the factor analytic sample in a stratified manner (i.e., random selection was constrained to conform with proportions of regional and ethnic distribution). The resulting normative sample closely matched U.S. Census distributions for region (see Table 3.2) with the exception of the Western part of the United States, which was somewhat underrepresented in the sample (i.e., 16.5% in the sample versus 21% in the Census). African-Americans were slightly overrepresented (18.5% in the sample versus 12% in the Census) in the normative group. Nevertheless, differences between sample proportions and U.S. Census data are minimal; thus, we consider the normative sample to be an adequate, representative sample of the U.S. child population.

Development of Normative Data: Results

ADHD Rating Scale–IV: Home Version

Normative data for parent ratings are provided separately for boys and girls in Tables 3.3 and 3.4, respectively, because of gender differences obtained, as described later in this chapter. Within each table, means and standard deviations are provided for three

TABLE 3.2. Percentage of Participants in Normative Sample by Region and Ethnic Group for the ADHD Rating Scale–IV: School Version

	Percentage in sample	U.S. Census percentage[a]
Region		
Northeast	20.0	20.0
Midwest	29.5	24.0
South	34.0	34.0
West	16.5	21.0
Ethnic group		
White, non-Latino	65.1	74.8
African-American	18.5	11.9
Latino	8.0	9.5
Native American	0.2	0.7
Asian-American	1.7	3.1
Other/missing	6.6	—

Note. From DuPaul et al. (1997). Copyright 1997 by the American Psychological Association. Reprinted by permission.
[a]Percentages are from 1990 U.S. Census data.

TABLE 3.3. Normative Data for Boys on the ADHD Rating Scale–IV: Home Version

Age (years)	n	Inattention					Hyperactivity–Impulsivity					Total score				
		M (SD)	80th %ile	90th %ile	93rd %ile	98th %ile	M (SD)	80th %ile	90th %ile	93rd %ile	98th %ile	M (SD)	80th %ile	90th %ile	93rd %ile	98th %ile
5–7	353	5.94 (5.08)	9.0	13.0	15.0	20.0	6.59 (5.56)	11.0	15.0	17.0	22.0	12.54 (9.97)	19.0	29.0	30.2	38.9
8–10	289	6.65 (5.33)	11.0	14.0	15.0	22.2	5.53 (5.25)	9.0	13.0	15.0	21.2	12.18 (9.81)	20.0	25.0	27.0	42.2
11–13	149	6.70 (6.27)	10.0	18.0	18.5	24.0	4.79 (5.54)	8.0	14.0	16.0	21.0	11.50 (11.32)	19.0	31.0	34.0	47.0
14–18	133	5.70 (5.36)	9.0	13.6	15.6	23.0	3.68 (4.32)	7.0	10.0	11.0	16.3	9.38 (8.96)	16.2	23.4	27.0	36.3

Note. From DuPaul, Anastopoulos, et al. (1998). Copyright 1998 by Plenum Publishing Corporation. Reprinted by permission.

TABLE 3.4. Normative Data for Girls on the ADHD Rating Scale–IV: Home Version

Age (years)	n	Inattention					Hyperactivity–Impulsivity					Total score				
		M (SD)	80th %ile	90th %ile	93rd %ile	98th %ile	M (SD)	80th %ile	90th %ile	93rd %ile	98th %ile	M (SD)	80th %ile	90th %ile	93rd %ile	98th %ile
5–7	314	4.51 (4.45)	7.0	10.0	12.0	18.0	5.00 (4.53)	8.0	11.0	13.0	19.7	9.51 (8.17)	15.0	20.5	24.0	30.0
8–10	327	4.17 (4.36)	7.0	10.0	12.0	16.4	3.39 (3.79)	6.0	8.0	9.0	15.4	7.56 (7.51)	12.0	16.2	20.0	30.4
11–13	173	4.61 (5.12)	8.0	11.0	12.8	21.0	2.88 (3.48)	5.0	7.6	9.0	12.0	7.49 (7.84)	13.0	18.0	20.0	28.5
14–18	225	4.07 (4.57)	7.0	11.0	12.2	16.5	3.29 (3.82)	5.0	8.0	10.0	16.0	7.36 (7.74)	12.0	19.0	22.0	32.5

Note. From DuPaul, Anastopoulos, et al. (1998). Copyright 1998 by Plenum Publishing Corporation. Reprinted by permission.

scores in accordance with factor analytic results: Inattention (sum of nine odd-numbered items), Hyperactivity–Impulsivity (sum of nine even-numbered items), and Total score (sum of Inattention and Hyperactivity–Impulsivity scores). Given the age differences in parent ratings (as described in a following section), separate normative data are provided for four age groups (5- to 7-year-olds, 8- to 10-year-olds, 11- to 13-year-olds, and 14- to 18-year-olds). Because very few cases were available for 4-, 19-, and 20-year-olds, these ages were not included in the normative data set. Although ethnic differences in parent ratings were obtained (as described later), normative data were not presented by ethnic group because there were insufficient numbers of participants for normative data to be displayed by gender, age, and ethnic group. Scores are provided for four cutoff points: 80th, 90th, 93rd, and 98th percentiles.

ADHD Rating Scale–IV: School Version

Normative data for teacher ratings are provided separately for boys and girls in Tables 3.5 and 3.6, respectively. Within each table, means and standard deviations are provided for three scores in accordance with factor analytic results: Inattention (sum of nine odd-numbered items), Hyperactivity–Impulsivity (sum of nine even-numbered items), and Total score (sum of Inattention and Hyperactivity–Impulsivity scores). Given the age differences obtained in teacher ratings (as described later), separate normative data are provided for four age groups (5- to 7-year-olds, 8- to 10-year-olds, 11- to 13-year-olds, and 14- to 18-year-olds). Because very few cases were available for 4- and 19-year-olds, these ages were not included in the normative data set. Separate norms for each ethnic group are not provided, because cell sizes (Sex × Age × Ethnic

TABLE 3.5. Normative Data for Boys on the ADHD Rating Scale–IV: School Version

Age (years)	n	Inattention					Hyperactivity–Impulsivity					Total score				
		M (SD)	80th %ile	90th %ile	93rd %ile	98th %ile	M (SD)	80th %ile	90th %ile	93rd %ile	98th %ile	M (SD)	80th %ile	90th %ile	93rd %ile	98th %ile
5–7	243	8.75 (7.66)	16.0	21.0	22.0	26.1	8.12 (7.86)	16.0	20.0	22.0	27.0	16.87 (14.61)	30.2	39.0	41.0	51.0
8–10	307	10.33 (8.49)	19.0	24.0	25.0	27.0	8.43 (8.05)	16.0	22.2	25.0	27.0	18.76 (15.51)	34.0	44.2	46.0	52.8
11–13	221	9.33 (8.11)	17.0	22.8	24.0	27.0	5.96 (6.72)	12.0	17.0	18.0	24.6	15.28 (13.55)	28.0	35.8	37.9	49.1
14–18	223	8.25 (7.27)	15.0	19.6	21.3	26.5	4.37 (6.09)	8.0	13.0	17.3	21.0	12.62 (12.16)	23.0	31.0	34.0	44.0

Note. From DuPaul et al. (1997). Copyright 1997 by the American Psychological Association. Reprinted by permission.

TABLE 3.6. Normative Data for Girls on the ADHD Rating Scale–IV: School Version

Age (years)	n	Inattention					Hyperactivity–Impulsivity					Total score				
		M (SD)	80th %ile	90th %ile	93rd %ile	98th %ile	M (SD)	80th %ile	90th %ile	93rd %ile	98th %ile	M (SD)	80th %ile	90th %ile	93rd %ile	98th %ile
5–7	211	6.59 (7.26)	13.0	19.0	21.0	24.0	5.66 (7.27)	11.0	18.8	21.1	25.8	12.25 (13.61)	23.0	36.0	40.0	46.8
8–10	258	6.04 (7.29)	10.2	19.0	21.0	26.0	3.81 (6.15)	6.2	12.0	16.7	25.0	9.86 (12.63)	16.0	30.2	34.9	50.0
11–13	222	5.97 (6.76)	11.4	17.0	19.0	24.0	3.62 (5.61)	6.4	10.7	14.8	23.5	9.59 (11.42)	17.0	27.0	31.4	42.1
14–18	216	4.09 (5.26)	8.0	13.0	14.8	18.0	1.97 (3.40)	3.0	8.0	9.0	12.7	6.06 (7.94)	11.0	18.3	21.8	27.7

Note. From DuPaul et al. (1997). Copyright 1997 by the American Psychological Association. Reprinted by permission.

Group) would be too small and because further research is necessary prior to the presentation of ethnic group norms. Scores are provided for four cutoff points: the 80th, 90th, 93rd, and 98th percentiles.

Sex, Age, and Ethnic Group Differences

ADHD Rating Scale–IV: Home Version

For the purposes of these analyses, three scores from the ADHD Rating Scale–IV: Home Version were used, including Inattention, Hyperactivity–Impulsivity, and Total. A 2 (Sex) × 4 (Age) × 3 (Ethnic Group) multivariate analysis of variance (MANOVA) was conducted, employing the three scores as the dependent variables. To maximize individual cell size, data for 4-, 19-, and 20-year-olds were dropped and the Age factor was blocked into four levels (5- to 7-year-olds, 8- to 10-year-olds, 11- to 13-year-olds, and 14- to 18-year-olds). Given the relatively small numbers of Asian-American and Native American participants, analyses of the effects of Ethnic group were restricted to Caucasian, African-American, and Latino children.

No statistically significant interactions were obtained. Statistically significant results were obtained for the main effects of Sex (Wilk's lambda = .99, $F(3, 4349)$ = 6.82, $p < .001$), Age (Wilk's lambda = .99, $F(9, 10584.47)$ = 5.96, $p < .001$), and Ethnic Group (Wilk's lambda = .99, $F(6, 8698)$ = 4.87, $p < .001$).

Separate 2 (Sex) × 4 (Age) × 3 (Ethnic Group) univariate analyses of variance (ANOVAs) were conducted for each of the ADHD Rating Scale–IV scores. A single significant interaction effect was obtained for Sex × Age for Hyperactivity–Impulsivity scores only ($F(3, 4351)$ = 3.10, $p < .05$). Simple effects tests of Age at each level of Sex, followed by Tukey Honestly Significant Difference (HSD) posthoc comparisons, were then conducted. Significant Age effects on Hyperactivity–Impulsivity scores were found for both boys ($F(3, 2166)$ = 46.44, $p < .001$) and girls ($F(3, 2498)$ = 35.16, $p < .001$). For both boys and girls, the youngest age group (5- to 7-year-olds) received higher ratings of Hyperactivity–Impulsivity symptoms than the three older age groups. Moreover, 8- to 10-year-old boys and girls received higher parent ratings than did the 11- to 13-year-olds. Finally, boys in the 8- to 10-year-old group received higher ratings than 14- to 18-year-old boys. No further age differences were found for girls. The pattern of age differences in parent-reported Hyperactivity–Impulsivity symptoms for boys and girls is portrayed in Figure 3.1. Boys were reported to exhibit more Hyperactivity–Impulsivity symptoms than girls for all age groups, except for 14- to 18-year-olds, in which mean scores were equivalent for boys and girls.

Significant main effects for Sex were found for Inattention ($F(1, 4351)$ = 12.93, $p < .001$), Hyperactivity–Impulsivity ($F(1, 4351)$ = 5.77, $p < .05$), and Total scores ($F(1, 4351)$ = 8.09, $p < .01$). Boys received higher ratings for ADHD symptoms than girls in all three cases. In similar fashion, significant main effects for Age were obtained for

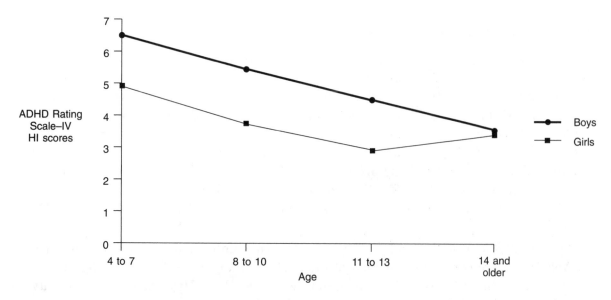

FIGURE 3.1. ADHD Rating Scale–IV: Home Version Hyperactivity–Impulsivity scores for boys and girls as a function of age. From DuPaul, Anastopoulos, et al. (1998). Copyright 1998 by Plenum Publishing Corporation. Reprinted by permission.

Inattention ($F(3, 4351) = 2.65$, $p < .05$), Hyperactivity–Impulsivity ($F(3, 4351) = 11.76$, $p < .001$), and Total scores ($F(3, 4351) = 5.40$, $p < .01$). Tukey HSD posthoc comparisons revealed that 11- to 13- and 14- to 18-year-olds received significantly lower Hyperactivity–Impulsivity and Total scores than did the two younger age groups. In similar fashion, 8- to 10-year-olds received lower Hyperactivity–Impulsivity and Total symptom ratings than did children in the 5- to 7-year-old age group. Fewer age differences were found for ratings of Inattention symptoms, wherein 14- to 18-year-olds received lower ratings than did 5- to 7- and 8- to 10-year-olds.

Significant main effects for Ethnic group were found for Inattention ($F(2, 4351) = 11.00$, $p < .001$), Hyperactivity–Impulsivity ($F(2, 4351) = 9.90$, $p < .001$), and Total scores ($F(2, 4351) = 11.95$, $p < .001$). Tukey HSD tests indicated that African-American participants received higher ratings on all three ADHD Rating Scale–IV scores than did Caucasian subjects, with no differences between Latino participants and the other two groups. Because correlations between parent ratings and Hollingshead Index scores (i.e., socioeconomic status) were significant (for Hyperactivity–Impulsivity $r = -.14$, $p < .001$; for Inattention $r = -.11$, $p < .001$), Ethnic Group effects were also examined using the Hollingshead Index as a covariate. Separate analyses of covariance indicated significant effects for Ethnic Group on Hyperactivity–Impulsivity ($F(2, 4119) = 3.92$, $p < .02$), Inattention ($F(2, 4119) = 7.46$, $p < .001$), and Total scores. ($F(2, 4119) = 6.92$, $p < .001$). The same pattern of between-group differences were evident, with African-American children receiving significantly higher ratings than Caucasian participants.

ADHD Rating Scale–IV: School Version

A 2 (Sex) × 4 (Age) × 3 (Ethnic Group) multivariate analysis of variance (MANOVA) was conducted employing the three ADHD Rating Scale--IV: School Version scores as the dependent variables. To maximize individual cell size, the Age factor was blocked into four levels (5- to 7-year-olds, 8- to 10-year-olds, 11- to 13-year-olds, and 14- to 18-year-olds). Given the relatively small numbers of Asian-American and Native American participants, the effects of Ethnic Group were examined only for Caucasian, African-American, and Latino children. Statistically significant results were obtained for the main effects of Sex (Wilk's lambda = .98, $F(3, 3569)$ = 30.25, p < .0001), Age (Wilk's lambda = .99, $F(9, 8686.16)$ = 4.97, p < .001), and Ethnic Group (Wilk's lambda = .96, $F(6, 7138)$ = 21.13, p < .0001).

Separate 2 (Sex) × 4 (Age) × 3 (Ethnic Group) univariate analyses of variance (ANOVAs) were conducted for each of the ADHD Rating Scale--IV scores. Significant interaction effects for Age × Ethnic Group were found for Hyperactivity--Impulsivity ($F(6, 3649)$ = 3.55, p < .01), and Total scores ($F(6, 3649)$ = 3.44, p < .01). Simple effects tests of Ethnic Group at each level of Age, followed by Tukey HSD posthoc comparisons, were then conducted. Significant Ethnic Group effects were found for both ADHD Rating Scale--IV scores within all four age groups (ps < .001). In the 5- to 7-year-old group, African-Americans received higher Hyperactivity--Impulsivity and

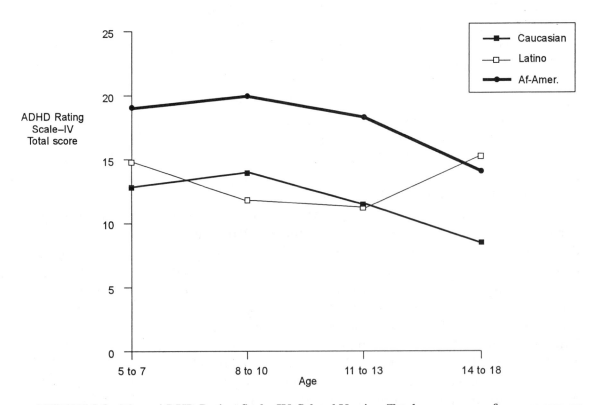

FIGURE 3.2. Mean ADHD Rating Scale--IV: School Version Total score across four age groups as a function of ethnic group. Af-Amer., African-American. From DuPaul et al. (1997). Copyright 1997 by the American Psychological Association. Reprinted by permission.

Total score ratings than Caucasians, with no other between-group differences. This pattern of Ethnic Group differences also was found within the 8- to 10-year-old and 11- to 13-year-old age groups. Further, African-Americans received higher ratings than did Latino participants in these latter two age ranges. Alternatively, both African-American and Latino adolescents in the 14- to 18-year-old group received higher ADHD ratings than Caucasians. To further illustrate these findings, the pattern of Ethnic Group differences in Total score across age groups is portrayed in Figure 3.2.

Significant main effects for Sex were found for Inattention ($F(1, 3571) = 76.12$, $p < .0001$), Hyperactivity--Impulsivity ($F(1, 3571) = 78.80$, $p < .0001$), and Total scores ($F(1, 3571) = 87.48$, $p < .0001$). Boys received higher ratings of ADHD symptoms than girls for Hyperactivity--Impulsivity and Total scores. A significant main effect for Age was obtained for Hyperactivity--Impulsivity scores only ($F(3, 3571) = 7.54$, $p < .0001$). Tukey HSD posthoc comparisons revealed that 14- to 18-year-olds received significantly lower ratings of Hyperactivity--Impulsivity symptoms than the three younger age groups. In similar fashion, 11- to 13-year-olds received lower Hyperactivity--Impulsivity ratings than children in the 5- to 7- and 8- to 10-year-old age groups. Finally, significant main effects for Ethnic Group were found for Inattention ($F(2, 3571) = 49.27$, $p < .0001$), Hyperactivity--Impulsivity ($F(2, 3571) = 58.44$, $p < .0001$), and Total scores ($F(2, 3571) = 59.25$, $p < .001$). Tukey HSD tests indicated that African-American participants received higher ratings on all three ADHD Rating Scale--IV scores than did Caucasian and Latino participants, with no differences between the latter two groups.

Summary of Sex, Age, and Ethnic Group Differences

Parent and teacher ratings of ADHD symptoms were found to vary significantly as a function of the sex, age, and ethnic group of the children being rated. As has been found in previous research, boys were reported to exhibit more frequent inattentive and hyperactive--impulsive behaviors than girls. Further, as has been the case in prior investigations, younger children received higher ratings of ADHD symptoms than older children. Given these results, we have presented normative data broken down by gender and age. Thus, a child undergoing an evaluation can be compared against norms based on that child's gender and age.

African-American children were rated by both parents and teachers to exhibit more frequent ADHD-related behaviors than were Caucasian and Latino children. This finding also is consistent with prior investigations of ethnic group differences. Interestingly, this group difference was maintained even when the effects of socioeconomic status were statistically removed. At present, it is unclear as to what factors might account for these group differences. Further, we are unable to provide separate norms for each ethnic group owing to insufficient cell size within gender and age groups. Thus, although our normative data are representative of the U.S. population in respect to ethnic group, clinicians should be cautious in using these data when evaluating African-American children so as to avoid overidentification of them as children with ADHD.

Epidemiology of ADHD Subtypes

Overall Prevalence

In view of the many circumstances that can affect the outcome of epidemiological research (e.g., method and source of symptom estimates), it is no wonder that there has been a tremendous amount of variability in the ADHD prevalence estimates that have been reported in the literature. For example, among the many studies utilizing DSM-III and DSM-III-R conceptualizations of ADHD, prevalence rates have ranged from as low as 2 to 3% up to 25 to 30% of the general child population. Whether this same pattern holds true for the DSM-IV version of ADHD is unclear, owing to the fact that relatively little research has thus far addressed this matter.

Using the normative samples described earlier in this chapter, we sought to determine prevalence rates of ADHD using DSM-IV criteria. For any given child, a symptom was considered present if the item score was a 2 or 3 (i.e., reported to occur often or very often, respectively). Conversely, item scores of 0 or 1 were indicative of symptom absence. Using the symptomatic cutoffs recommended in DSM-IV (i.e., six of nine symptoms of inattention, and/or six of nine symptoms of hyperactivity--impulsivity), the number of children meeting criteria for each of the three subtypes of ADHD was determined. Given these assumptions, we found an overall ADHD prevalence rate of 7.5% based on parent ratings on the Home Version and a prevalance rate of 21.6% based on teacher ratings on the School Version. These estimates of overall disorder are commensurate with prevalence rates obtained in other recent investigations using DSM-IV criteria and *a single informant* (e.g., Gaub & Carlson, 1997; Wolraich, Hannah, Pinnock, Baumgaertel, & Brown, 1996). It should be noted that prevalence estimates are likely to be *upper-bound estimates,* because these are based on symptom frequency counts alone and on the report of a single informant and, therefore, *should be interpreted with caution.*

In terms of subtyping considerations, the Combined category was the one that emerged most often in the DSM-IV clinical field trials, outnumbering the Inattentive and Hyperactive--Impulsive subgroups on the order of 2:1 and 3:1, respectively (Lahey et al., 1994). Perhaps because of the nonclinical nature of the samples we employed, our estimates of subtype prevalence are discrepant with the field trial results. In particular, we found the Inattentive subtype to be most prevalent in our samples. Specifically, teacher ratings on the School Version indicated a prevalence of 10% for the Inattentive subtype, 3.2% for the Hyperactive--Impulsive subtype, and 8.4% for the Combined subtype. The same pattern was also evident when parents served as informants, with rates of 3.2%, 2.1%, and 2.2% occurring for the Inattentive, Hyperactive--Impulsive, and Combined subtypes, respectively.

Age and Gender Effects on Prevalence

When viewed from the perspective of clinical practice, these results are of limited significance, because they do not shed light on individual differences. Of the many individual difference variables that may be considered, age and gender are certainly among those that can have a powerful influence on child psychopathology prevalence estimates.

Teacher ratings on the School Version resulted in overall prevalence rates of 25.3% for children 5 to 7 years of age, 23.8% for 8- to 10-year-old children, 21.5% for the 11- to 13-year-olds, and 15.0 % for those 14 to 18 years of age. When parents served as informants, the overall prevalence rates were 9.1% for 5- to 7-year-old children, 6.4% for 8- to 10-year-old children, 8.3% for 11- to 13-year-old children, and 5.8% for adolescents between 14 and 18 years of age. These results raise the possibility that the overall prevalence of ADHD, as defined by DSM-IV symptom frequency criteria, declines with age.

As shown in Table 3.7, developmental trends also appear to be evident among the various subtyping categories, but the exact manner in which they unfold seems to vary as a function of the informant. For example, teacher ratings have suggested that children 5 to 10 years of age are much more likely to be identified with the Combined subtype, followed in order by the Inattentive and Hyperactive--Impulsive subtypes. For students 11 to 18 years of age the picture changes somewhat, with the Inattentive subtype becoming the most prevalent, followed in order by the Combined and Hyperactive--Impulsive classifications. In contrast, parent ratings have suggested that the Hyperactive--Impulsive subtype occurs more often than the other two major subtyping categories among children 5 to 7 years of age. That this subtyping category would be so prevalent among younger children is by no means unusual, as it has also been reported by other investigators, including those using clinical samples (Lahey et al., 1994). For reasons that are not entirely clear, the prevalence of the Hyperactive--Impulsive subtype decreases dramatically among children 8 years of age and older, making it the least likely subtype to occur in this age group. For these same children

TABLE 3.7. Prevalence of ADHD across Development in a Community Sample

Informant	Age group				Total
	5--7 years	8--10 years	11--13 years	14--17 years	
Parents					
Overall	9.1%	6.4%	8.3%	5.8%	7.5%
By subtype	HI > C > I	I > C > HI	I > C > HI	I > C > HI	I > C > HI
Teachers					
Overall	25.3%	23.8%	21.5%	15.0%	21.6%
By subtype	C > I > HI	C > I > HI	I > C > HI	I > C > HI	I > C > HI

Note. C, Combined subtype; I, Predominantly Inattentive subtype; HI, Predominantly Hyperactive--Impulsive subtype.

and adolescents, the prevalence of the Inattentive category increases, thereby making it the most frequently encountered subtyping classification.

Implicit throughout the preceding discussion is the notion that ADHD changes in its clinical presentation across development. Although this may seem to be a reasonable conclusion, these findings were derived from cross-sectional investigations. Whether these same developmental trends would be evident in longitudinal studies is unknown. Until research of this sort is completed, there are at least cross-sectional data available to raise the possibility that developmental trends exist.

Along with these age-related effects, gender can also influence not only the overall rate of ADHD, but the relative prevalence of each subtype. Specifically, parent ratings on the Home Version indicated a ratio of boys to girls of 1.4:1 for the Inattentive subtype, 3.1:1 for the Hyperactive--Impulsive subtype, and 3.3:1 for the Combined subtype. A similar pattern of findings emerged from the teacher ratings, with ratios of 2:1 for the Inattentive subtype, 3.2:1 for the Hyperactive--Impulsive subtype, and 2.6:1 for the Combined subtype.

Ethnic Group Differences

In the DSM-IV clinical field trials, ethnicity was not a major factor influencing the prevalence of ADHD (Lahey et al., 1994). Ethnicity did, however, appear to have an impact on our findings with a community-based sample. Teacher ratings on the School Version identified approximately 6.3% of the Caucasian children and adolescents as having one of the three major subtypes of ADHD versus a rate of 12.3% among children and adolescents from minority backgrounds (i.e., African-American and Latino). Looking at it from a somewhat different perspective, we can say that of the total number of children and adolescents identified with any type of ADHD, 43.4% were from minority backgrounds, even though minority children and adolescents made up only 34.8% of the total teacher-generated sample. Similar findings emerged from parent ratings on the Home Version. Unfortunately, very little of the ADHD research that has been published to date has addressed ethnic diversity issues. Additional research of this type is clearly needed to establish a more definitive connection between ethnicity and the prevalence of ADHD. Pending the results of further investigations, clinicians should employ caution in using these scales to diagnose children and adolescents from minority backgrounds.

Summary of Prevalence Rates

Prevalence rates derived from our normative samples are higher than the 3 to 5% prevalence described in DSM-IV. This should not be surprising, given that our rates were derived primarily on the basis of the ADHD symptom frequency requirement alone and the report of a single informant. Having been determined in this way, such figures very likely include many children for whom ADHD would not be diagnosed, owing to the fact that they would not meet all of the other DSM-IV criteria (e.g., impairment in functioning, age of onset prior to 7 years old, and display of symptoms across more than one setting). In light of these circumstances, our estimates are perhaps best viewed as *upper limits* in the true prevalence of ADHD within the general population.

Among clinic samples, the Combined subtype appears to be the most commonly encountered subtype category (Lahey et al., 1994), whereas the Inattentive subtype occurs most often in community samples, as presented here. Such a difference suggests that a more severe ADHD presentation is what prompts parents and teachers to refer a child for clinical services. Conversely, this also raises the possibility that many children with milder forms of ADHD are not receiving services, which potentially may serve to decrease their risk for encountering more serious problems. In addition to these referral considerations, many other factors may affect the prevalence of these subtypes. According to teachers, younger children display the Combined subtype most often, whereas older children and adolescents are much more likely to be identified with the Inattentive classification. Similar findings have emerged from parent ratings of older children and adolescents (see Barkley, 1998), but parents are much more likely to identify very young children as having the Hyperactive--Impulsive subtype consistent with the DSM-IV field trials. Of additional interest is that the overall prevalence of DSM-IV defined ADHD—that is, the total for all three major subtypes—seems to decline with age. Although these findings certainly point to the existence of developmental trends, such a conclusion is limited by the fact that it is based on investigations utilizing cross-sectional, rather than longitudinal, designs.

CHAPTER 4

Reliability and Validity

In this chapter, we review the psychometric properties and technical adequacy of the Home and School Versions of the ADHD Rating Scale–IV. First, a brief description of the samples and procedures used to conduct these analyses is provided. Then, data regarding the internal consistency, test–retest reliability, interrater agreement, criterion-related validity, and discriminant validity of both versions of the scale are presented. Finally, to shed further light on the clinical utility of these scales, data are presented on the predictive validity of ADHD Rating Scale–IV scores in the context of clinic-based and school-based evaluations.

Sample and Procedures: Reliability and Criterion-Related Validity

Participants

The sample consisted of 71 students (35 boys, 36 girls) ranging in age from 5 to 17 years ($M = 11.0$; $SD = 3.4$) and was randomly selected from two suburban school districts located in eastern Pennsylvania and southern New Jersey (DuPaul, Power, McGoey, Ikeda, & Anastopoulos, 1998). Participants were predominantly Caucasian ($n = 60$) but also included children of African-American ($n = 5$), Latino ($n = 4$), and Asian-American ($n = 2$) backgrounds. This sample was used to examine the test–retest reliability, internal consistency, and criterion-related validity of ADHD ratings.

Teacher Ratings

Complete data for analyzing the test–retest reliability of teacher ratings were available for 52 children (24 boys, 28 girls) ranging in age from 5 to 17 years ($M = 11.3$; $SD = 3.6$) who attended kindergarten through 12th grade ($M = 5.7$; $SD = 3.7$). For the validity analyses of teacher ratings, three of the criterion measures involved direct observation of classroom behavior for a subsample of 53 students (25 boys, 28 girls) ranging in age from 5 to 14 years ($M = 9.8$; $SD = 2.6$) who attended kindergarten through eighth grade ($M = 4.0$; $SD = 2.6$).

Parent Ratings

Complete test–retest reliability data for parent ratings were available for 43 children (17 boys, 26 girls) ranging in age from 5 to 17 years ($M = 11.07$; $SD = 3.50$) who attended kindergarten through 12th grade ($M = 5.35$; $SD = 3.59$). For the validity analyses, three of the criterion measures involved direct observation of classroom behavior for a subsample of 46 students (22 boys, 24 girls) ranging in age from 5 to 14 years ($M = 10.09$; $SD = 2.58$) who attended kindergarten through eighth grade ($M = 4.30$; $SD = 2.62$).

Interobserver Agreement

For analysis of interobserver agreement, parent and teacher ratings were available for a sample of 62 students (28 boys, 34 girls). These students ranged in age from 5 to 17 years ($M = 11.1$; $SD = 3.4$) and attended kindergarten through 12th grade ($M = 5.4$; $SD = 3.5$).

Measures

Parents and teachers were asked to provide information about the child being rated, such as gender, grade, and age. Teachers completed the ADHD Rating Scale–IV: School Version and the Conners Teacher Rating Scale–39 (CTRS-39; Conners, 1989). Parents completed the ADHD Rating Scale–IV: Home Version and the Conners Parent Rating Scale–48 (CPRS-48; Conners, 1989).

The classroom behavior of children who were placed in kindergarten through eighth grade was observed by a research assistant using an adaptation of the ADHD Behavior Code originally designed by Barkley (1990). The occurrence of two behaviors (i.e., Off-Task and Fidgets) was recorded on a partial interval basis using observation intervals of 10 seconds with 5 seconds between intervals used for recording observed behaviors. "Off-Task" behavior was defined as the student's breaking eye contact with task materials or classroom instruction for at least 3 consecutive seconds. "Fidgets" was defined as purposeless motion of the legs, arms, hands, buttocks, or trunk that occurred at least four times in succession. Each observation session was approximately 15 minutes in length. For each behavior, the percentage of intervals in which the behavior occurred was calculated by dividing the number of intervals in which the behavior occurred by the total number of observation intervals and multiplying the dividend by 100%.

An academic efficiency score (AES; Rapport, DuPaul, & Kelly, 1989) was calculated for each participant who was observed in the classroom. For each student, teachers submitted three samples of independent seat work completed in the classroom. The AES was calculated by dividing the number of work items correctly completed by the number of items assigned and multiplying the dividend by 100%. This score represented the quality of each child's academic performance in relation to his or her classmates, who were presumably asked to complete the same amount of work at similar levels of difficulty.

Procedures

Parent and teacher ratings were obtained over a 1-month period in May and June 1995 (to ensure teacher familiarity with student behavior). Within each of the two districts, two to four children (with an attempt to include equivalent numbers of boys and girls) at each grade level were randomly selected to participate. Only children in general education classrooms participated.

Once written parental permission was obtained, parents and teachers were asked to complete the appropriate version of the ADHD Rating Scale–IV on two occasions 4 weeks apart to assess test–retest reliability. On each occasion, ratings were completed on Fridays and were to reflect observations of the child's behavior over the previous week. The CTRS-39 was also completed by the teacher on one of the two occasions, and the CPRS-48 was completed by the parent on one of the two occasions. For all children in kindergarten through eighth grade, a research assistant conducted behavioral observations on three separate days (i.e., a total of 45 minutes of observation) during 1 of the 2 weeks when parents and teachers were due to complete the ADHD Rating Scale–IV. Following each observation, the teacher provided information necessary to calculate an AES score (i.e., how much work was completed correctly relative to the amount assigned). A second observer was present for 30% of the observation sessions so that interobserver agreement could be determined. Interobserver agreement was calculated by dividing the number of agreements by the total number of agreements plus disagreements and multiplying the dividend by 100%. Agreement was consistently above 80% and averaged 88% across the two behavioral categories.

Internal Consistency, Reliability, and Interobserver Agreement

Coefficient alphas were calculated to determine the internal consistency of the ADHD Rating Scale–IV: School Version and its two subscales. The following alpha coefficients were obtained: Total score = .94, Inattention = .96, and Hyperactivity–Impulsivity = .88. Test–retest reliability data were obtained for teacher ratings occurring 4 weeks apart. Pearson product–moment correlation coefficients were as follows: Total score = .90, Inattention = .89, and Hyperactivity–Impulsivity = .88.

In similar fashion, coefficient alphas were calculated to determine the internal consistency of the ADHD Rating Scale–IV: Home Version and its two subscales. The following alpha coefficients were obtained: Total score = .92, Inattention = .86, and Hyperactivity–Impulsivity = .88. Test–retest reliability data were obtained for parent ratings occurring 4 weeks apart. Pearson product–moment correlation coefficients were as follows: Total score = .85, Inattention = .78, and Hyperactivity–Impulsivity = .86. Interrater agreement coefficients between parents and teachers were in the moderate range, as follows: Total score = .41, Inattention = .45, and Hyperactivity– Impulsivity = .40.

Relationships between Teacher ADHD Ratings and Criterion Measures

Pearson product–moment correlations between ADHD Rating Scale–IV: School Version scores and criterion measures (i.e., CTRS-39 scores, direct observations of off-task and fidgety behavior, and mean AES) are presented in Table 4.1. Overall, the absolute values of obtained Pearson correlation coefficients ranged from .22 to .88, with 28 out of 30 achieving statistical significance. If a Bonferroni correction is applied to control Type 1 error rate for multiple correlations (i.e., $\alpha = .002$), 20 of these correlations can be considered statistically significant. As expected, the strongest correlations were found between ADHD Rating Scale–IV: School Version factor scores and CTRS-39 Hyperactivity and Hyperactivity Index scores. In fact, ratings of ADHD symptoms on these two measures shared between 53 and 77% of the variance. The correlation between the Hyperactivity–Impulsivity subscale and CTRS-39 Conduct Problems was significantly greater than the correlation between the Inattention subscale and Conduct Problems ($t(70) = 2.54$, $p < .01$). Conversely, the correlations between the Inattention subscale and CTRS-39 Anxious–Passive and Daydreams–Attention scales were significantly greater than the correlations between these two CTRS-39 scales and the Hyperactivity–Impulsivity subscale ($t(70) = 1.99$, $p < .05$; $t(70) = 6.13$, $p < .001$, respectively). No other significant differences between the Inattention and Hyperactivity–Impulsivity subscales were obtained.

The ADHD Rating Scale–IV: School Version Total score and Inattention subscale score were significantly correlated with direct observations of classroom off-task and fidgety behavior (see Table 4.1). The correlations between the Hyperactivity–Impulsivity

TABLE 4.1. Validity Coefficients for ADHD Rating Scale–IV: School Version

Measure	Inattention	Hyperactivity–Impulsivity	Total
CTRS Hyperactivity[a]	.73***	.79***	.86***
CTRS Conduct Problems[a]	.29*	.55***	.44***
CTRS Emot-Indulgence[a]	.54***	.41**	.56***
CTRS Anxious–Passive[a]	.47***	.25*	.45***
CTRS Asocial[a]	.43***	.36***	.46***
CTRS Daydream–Att[a]	.85***	.44***	.80***
CTRS Hyper Index[a]	.76***	.76***	.88***
Mean Off-Task[b]	.35**	.22	.34**
Mean Fidgets[b]	.28*	.23	.29*
Mean Accuracy[b]	–.46***	–.34**	–.47***

Note. CTRS, Conners Teacher Rating Scale–39; Emot-Indulgence, Emotional Indulgence; Daydream–Att, Daydream–Attention Problems; Hyper Index, Hyperactivity Index. From DuPaul, Power, et al. (1998). Copyright 1998 by The Psychoeducational Corporation. Reprinted by permission.
[a]$n = 71$; [b]$n = 53$. *$p < .05$; **$p < .01$; ***$p < .001$.

subscale and classroom behavior were nonsignificant. All three ADHD Rating Scale–IV: School Version scores were significantly associated, in a negative fashion, with accuracy on academic tasks. It should be noted that correlations with classroom observation measures were lower than correlations with CTRS-39 ratings. In fact, only two of the nine correlations with observational measures were significant at the .002 alpha level. Higher teacher ratings of ADHD symptoms were associated with lower levels of task accuracy and, in the case of the Inattention subscale, higher frequencies of off-task and fidgety behavior.

Relationships between Parent ADHD Ratings and Criterion Measures

Pearson product–moment correlations between ADHD Rating Scale–IV: Home Version scores and CPRS-48 scores are presented in Table 4.2. Overall, the absolute values of obtained validity coefficients ranged from .10 to .81, with 15 out of 18 achieving statistical significance. If a Bonferroni correction is applied to control Type 1 error rate for multiple correlations (i.e., α = .003), 12 of these correlations can be considered statistically significant. As expected, the strongest correlations were found between ADHD Rating Scale–IV: Home Version and CPRS-48 Hyperactivity Index scores. In fact, ratings of ADHD symptoms on these two measures shared between 37 and 66% of the variance. The pattern of correlations provided initial evidence for the discriminant validity of the Inattention and Hyperactivity–Impulsivity subscales. Significantly stronger correlations were obtained between the Hyperactivity–Impulsivity subscale and the CPRS-48 Conduct Problems ($t(56)$ = 2.19, p < .05), Hyperactivity–Impulsivity ($t(56)$ = 4.65, p < .001), and Hyperactivity Index ($t(56)$ = 2.99, p < .01) scores than were found between the Inattention subscale and these three indices. Conversely, the Inattention subscale was more strongly correlated with the CPRS-48 Learning Problems scale than was the Hyperactivity–Impulsivity subscale ($t(56)$ = 2.44, p < .01). Neither ADHD Rating Scale–IV subscale correlated significantly with CPRS-48 Anxious ratings.

TABLE 4.2. Correlation Coefficients between Parent Ratings on the ADHD Rating Scale–IV: Home Version and Conners Parent Rating Scale–Revised

Measure	Inattention	Hyperactivity–Impulsivity	Total
CPRS Conduct Problems	.45***	.65***	.61***
CPRS Learning Problems	.66***	.45***	.60***
CPRS Psycho	.28*	.32**	.36**
CPRS Imp–Hyp	.45***	.78***	.68***
CPRS Anxious	.05	.18	.10
CPRS Hyper Index	.61***	.81***	.80***

Note. CPRS, Conners Parent Rating Scale-48; Psycho, Psychosomatic; Imp–Hyp, Impulsivity–Hyperactivity. n = 43. From DuPaul, Power, et al. (1998). Copyright 1998 by The Psychoeducational Corporation. Reprinted by permission.

*p < .05; **p < .01; ***p < .001.

TABLE 4.3. Correlations between Parent Ratings on the ADHD Rating Scale–IV: Home Version and School Behavior

Measure	Inattention	Hyperactivity–Impulsivity	Total
CTRS Anxious–Passive[a]	.18	.14	.20
CTRS Asocial[a]	.13	.14	.20
CTRS Conduct Problems[a]	.39**	.26*	.38**
CTRS Daydream–Att[a]	.32*	.18	.28*
CTRS Emot–Indulgence[a]	.15	−.02	.12
CTRS Hyperactivity[a]	.38**	.35**	.41**
CTRS Hyper Index[a]	.30*	.31*	.34*
Mean Off-Task[b]	.28	.14	.26
Mean Fidgets[b]	.15	.17	.25
Mean Accuracy[b]	−.43**	−.18	−.36**

Note. From DuPaul, Power, et al. (1998). Copyright 1998 by The Psychoeducational Corporation. Reprinted by permission.
[a]$n = 62$; [b]$n = 46$. *$p < .05$; **$p < .01$.

Parent ratings of ADHD symptoms were significantly correlated with teacher ratings on the CTRS-39 Hyperactivity and Conduct Problems factors as well as the Hyperactivity Index (see Table 4.3). In addition, parent Inattention and Total scores were correlated with the CTRS-39 Daydreams–Attention Problem factor. ADHD Rating Scale–IV: Home Version scores were not correlated with teacher ratings of anxious–passive, asocial, or emotionally indulgent behavior. Contrary to expectations, parent ratings were not significantly correlated with classroom observations of either off-task or fidgety behavior (see Table 4.3). Alternatively, both the Inattention subscale and Total scores were significantly associated, in a negative fashion, with accuracy on academic tasks. Thus, higher parent ratings of inattentive symptoms and Total score were associated with lower levels of task accuracy. It should be noted that the correlations between parent ratings and school validity data were relatively low, and with a Bonferroni correction ($\alpha = .002$), none of the obtained coefficients reached statistical significance.

Sample and Procedures: Discriminant Validity

Participants

This sample was used to examine the discriminant validity of parent and teacher ADHD ratings and consisted of consecutive referrals to the ADHD Evaluation and Treatment Program of the Children's Seashore House in Philadelphia. All children were referred for an initial evaluation or a reevaluation of ADHD. Participants met the following inclusion criteria: (1) completion by parents and teachers of the ADHD Rating Scale–IV and a diagnostic interview with parents using the Diagnostic Interview for Children and Adolescents–Revised (DICA-R; Reich, Shayka, & Taibleson, 1991) updated to reflect DSM-IV criteria (Eiraldi, Power, & Nezu, 1997); and (2) estimated

IQ of 80 or above on the Kaufman Brief Intelligence Test (KBIT; Kaufman & Kaufman, 1990). Children were excluded if they presented evidence of pervasive developmental disorder, a psychotic disorder, or a progressive neurological disorder. Children were also excluded if they took a psychotropic medication for ADHD or related disorders within 6 months of the time of evaluation.

The sample consisted of 92 children (24 girls, 68 boys) between the ages of 6 and 14.75 years ($M = 9.0$, $SD = 2.2$). Grade levels ranged from kindergarten through eighth grade, with 73% of the sample attending grades 1 through 4. The distribution of ethnic groups represented was 21.7% African-American, 3.3% Latino, and 75% Caucasian. The range of socioeconomic levels as assessed by the Four Factor Index of Social Status (Hollingshead, 1975) was as follows: 3.2% in Category I (unskilled laborers), 14.2% in Category II (machine operators, semiskilled workers), 25% in Category III (skilled craftsman, clerical, sales workers), 40.2% in Category IV (small business owners, technicians), and 17.4% in Category V (major business owners, professionals). On the KBIT, the sample achieved mean scores of 103.1 ($SD = 11.9$) on the Vocabulary scale, 100.5 ($SD = 11.7$) on Matrices, and 101.9 ($SD = 11.1$) on the Composite.

Procedures

Parents and teachers completed the Child Behavior Checklist (CBCL; Achenbach, 1991a, 1991b, 1991c), the teacher-rated Child Attention Problems scale (CAP; Barkley, 1990), and home and school versions of the ADHD Rating Scale–IV prior to their initial clinic visit. The DICA-R was conducted by a doctoral-level psychology clinician or an advanced doctoral candidate in psychology at the initial clinic visit.

Children were assigned to a diagnostic group or clinical control group on the basis of their scores on a multimethod assessment battery including the parent version of the DICA-R, the parent-rated CBCL, and the teacher-rated CAP. Children were categorized as having ADHD, Predominantly Inattentive subtype (ADHD/I) if they demonstrated the following: (1) a DICA-R diagnosis of ADHD/I, (2) a T score of 60 or above on the Attention Problems factor of the CBCL, and (3) a score on the Inattention subscale of the CAP of greater than or equal to the 93rd percentile. Children were diagnosed with ADHD, Combined subtype (ADHD/COM), if they demonstrated (1) a DICA-R diagnosis of ADHD/COM, (2) a T score of 60 or above on the Attention Problems factor of the CBCL, and (3) scores on the Inattention and Overactivity subscales of the CAP of greater than or equal to the 93rd percentile. Two children met the criteria for ADHD, Predominantly Hyperactive–Impulsive subtype, and were not included in further analyses. Remaining children who did not meet the criteria for any of the ADHD subtypes were assigned to a clinical control group.

Based on these criteria, 30 children were classified as having ADHD/I, 25 participants had ADHD/COM, and 35 children were assigned to the clinical control group. Although the ADHD/COM group had a higher proportion of participants with a comorbid conduct disorder, there were no further differences between groups in respect to psychiatric comorbidity, gender, age, or special education placement.

Discriminant Validity of Parent and Teacher Ratings

Means and standard deviations for parent and teacher Inattention and Hyperactivity–Impulsivity scores across three groups (ADHD/COM, ADHD/I, and clinical control) are presented in Table 4.4. Statistically significant differences in mean ratings between these three groups were obtained for parent Inattention ratings ($F(2, 87) = 7.56$, $p < .001$), parent Hyperactivity–Impulsivity ratings ($F(2, 87) = 5.60$, $p < .01$), teacher Inattention ratings ($F(2, 87) = 22.34$, $p < .0001$), and teacher Hyperactivity–Impulsivity ratings ($F(2, 87) = 23.57$, $p < .0001$). Tukey HSD post hoc comparisons (conducted using an alpha level of .05) indicated that parent and teacher Inattention ratings were significantly higher (indicating greater levels of inattention) for participants in the predominantly Inattentive and Combined subtype groups relative to clinical controls. Alternatively, parent and teacher Hyperactivity–Impulsivity ratings were significantly higher for participants in the Combined subtype group relative to their counterparts in the other two groups. There were no significant differences in parent and teacher Hyperactivity–Impulsivity scores between the predominantly Inattentive subtype and clinical control participants.

Predictive Validity

To further evaluate the validity of the ADHD Rating Scale–IV, we investigated the ability of this measure to differentiate children with ADHD from those without this disorder as well as to distinguish children with the two most common subtypes of

TABLE 4.4. Means and Standard Deviations of ADHD Rating Scale–IV Scores across Clinical Groups

Measure	Group		
	Control	ADHD/I	ADHD/COM
Parent Inattention	14.2 (7.9)[a]	19.3 (4.4)[b]	19.3 (4.3)[b]
Parent Hyperactivity–Impulsivity	11.6 (8.0)[a]	10.7 (5.7)[a]	16.4 (5.9)[b]
Teacher Inattention	13.3 (5.9)[a]	19.3 (4.7)[b]	21.6 (4.3)[b]
Teacher Hyperactivity–Impulsivity	10.5 (8.0)[a]	6.9 (4.5)[a]	18.6 (5.7)[b]

Note. ADHD/I, ADHD Predominantly Inattentive subtype; ADHD/COM, ADHD Combined subtype. Standard deviations are in parentheses. Means with different superscripts were significantly different at the $p < .05$ level. From DuPaul, Power, et al. (1998). Copyright 1998 by The Psychoeducational Corporation. Reprinted by permission.

ADHD, the Combined subtype (ADHD/COM) and the Inattentive subtype (ADHD/I). We conducted predictive validity studies in both a clinical and a school setting.

Prediction in a Clinical Setting

The sample and procedures for diagnosing participants in our clinic-based predictive validity study (see Power, Doherty, et al., 1998) were described in the previous section under "Sample and Procedures: Discriminant Validity."

Logistic regression methods were used to evaluate (1) whether parent and teacher ratings used separately were able to differentiate clinical groups from the control group, and clinical groups from each other and (2) whether a strategy combining parent and teacher ratings achieved a higher level of diagnostic accuracy than a single-informant approach. Logistic regression generates a correlation-type statistic (R) reflecting the unique association between each predictor variable and the criterion variable (i.e., diagnostic group membership), and a chi-square statistic indicating whether the logistic model results in a significant level of prediction and whether each additional variable entered into the model results in an improvement in prediction.

Predictive Validity of the Inattention Subscale

Table 4.5 presents the results of logistic regression analyses evaluating the ability of the Inattention subscale to differentiate children with ADHD/I from those in the control group. Both teacher ratings and parent ratings, when entered separately, were predictive of membership in the ADHD/I versus control group. The association between teacher ratings of Inattention and diagnostic status was moderate ($R = .38$), and the association between parent ratings of Inattention and diagnostic status was low ($R = .26$). In a forward stepwise logistic regression analysis, teacher ratings entered the equation first. The addition of parent ratings resulted in a significant improvement of the logistic model ($\chi^2 = 6.85$, $p < .01$). The combination of teacher and parent ratings

TABLE 4.5. Results of Logistic Regression Analyses When Using the Inattention Subscale: Clinic-Based Study

Comparison	χ^2	p	R	Prediction
ADHD/I versus control group				
Teacher ratings	18.68	.0001	.38	74%
Parent ratings	10.72	.0001	.26	68%
ADHD/COM versus control group				
Teacher ratings	24.11	.0001	.44	80%
Parent ratings	8.08	.005	.23	62%

in the model correctly classified 72% of the cases; however, this was slightly less than the percentage predicted by teacher ratings alone (74%).

Next, logistic regression analyses were used to evaluate the ability of the Inattention subscale to differentiate children with ADHD/COM from those in the control group (see Table 4.5). Once again, both teacher ratings and parent ratings, when entered separately, were predictive of membership in the ADHD/COM group versus the control group. The association between teacher ratings of Inattention and diagnostic status was moderate ($R = .44$). The use of teacher ratings alone correctly classified 80% of the participants. In contrast, the association between parent ratings of Inattention and diagnostic status was low ($R = .23$). In a forward stepwise logistic regression analysis, teacher ratings only entered the equation first; the addition of parent ratings did not result in a significant improvement of the logistic model.

Predictive Validity of the Hyperactivity–Impulsivity Subscale

Table 4.6 presents the results of logistic regression analyses used to evaluate the ability of the Hyperactivity–Impulsivity subscale to differentiate children with ADHD/COM from those in the control group. Both teacher ratings and parent ratings, when entered separately, were able to predict membership in the ADHD/COM versus control group. The association between teacher ratings of Hyperactivity–Impulsivity and diagnostic status was low to moderate ($R = .32$), and the association between parent ratings of Hyperactivity–Impulsivity and diagnostic status was low ($R = .22$). In a forward stepwise logistic regression analysis, teacher ratings entered the equation first. The addition of parent ratings resulted in significant improvement of the logistic model ($\chi^2(1) = 7.18$, $p < .01$). The combination of teacher and parent ratings in the model correctly classified 75% of the cases.

Next, logistic regression analyses were used to evaluate the ability of the Hyperactivity–Impulsivity subscale to differentiate children with ADHD/COM from those with

TABLE 4.6. Results of Logistic Regression Analyses When Using the Hyperactivity–Impulsivity Subscale: Clinic-Based Study

Comparison	χ^2	p	R	Prediction
ADHD/COM versus control group				
Teacher ratings	12.70	.001	.32	65%
Parent ratings	6.95	.01	.22	60%
ADHD/COM versus ADHD/I				
Teacher ratings	30.14	.0001	.46	84%
Parent ratings	7.69	.01	.24	64%

ADHD/I (see Table 4.6). Both teacher ratings and parent ratings, when entered separately, were able to predict membership in the ADHD/COM group versus the ADHD/I group. The association between teacher ratings of Hyperactivity–Impulsivity and diagnostic status was moderate ($R = .46$); teacher ratings correctly classified 84% of the cases. In contrast, the association between parent ratings of Hyperactivity–Impulsivity and diagnostic status was low ($R = .24$). In a forward stepwise logistic regression analysis, teacher ratings only entered the equation first; the addition of parent ratings failed to result in significant improvement of the logistic model.

Conclusions

Results from the clinic-based study demonstrated that the Inattention subscale was able to differentiate children with ADHD/I from a control group, and children with ADHD/COM from controls. In addition, logistic regression analyses indicated that the Hyperactivity–Impulsivity subscale successfully differentiated children with ADHD/COM from controls, and children with ADHD/COM from those with ADHD/I. The results revealed that teacher ratings on the ADHD Rating Scale–IV are extremely important in predicting subtype membership. Although parent ratings were also significantly predictive of diagnostic status, teacher ratings were better at predicting ADHD subtypes than parent ratings. Further, the results suggested that an approach to diagnostic prediction that includes both teachers and parents is often superior to a single informant approach.

Prediction in a School Setting

Participants in our school-based predictive validity study (see Power, Andrews, et al., in press) were referred students from two school districts, both of which served children in kindergarten through eighth grade. Participants were students in general education referred by their teachers to the school's Pupil Assistance Committee (PAC) for academic and/or behavioral problems. During the course of the study, 259 students were referred to PAC teams. Parents of students referred to PAC were sent a letter informing them about the study and requesting permission for their child to be screened for attention and behavior problems through the use of parent and teacher rating scales. One hundred fifty-six (60%) of the parents or guardians gave permission for their child to be screened. Nine students were excluded because they were taking medication, leaving 147 participants, 48 of whom were girls. Students ranged in age from 5 through 14 years, with a mean of 9 years. The ethnic groups represented were 29.6% African-American, 3.7% Latino, 1.2% Native American, 2.5% Asian-American, and 61.7% Caucasian. Almost 90% of the sample were in the middle categories of socioeconomic status.

A multigate screening process was used to determine which students met the criteria for ADHD. The parents of all students referred to PAC during the course of the study were sent a letter inviting them to participate in a screening to assess attention and behavior problems. Parents who gave consent were asked to complete the ADHD Rating Scale–IV for their referred child. In addition, students whose parents granted consent were rated by teachers on the Child Attention Profile (CAP) and ADHD Rating

Scale–IV. Students rated at or above the 93rd percentile on the Inattention and/or Overactivity factor of the CAP met screening criteria for ADHD and were advanced to the next stage of evaluation. Students who did not meet screening criteria were not assessed further. Ninety-five students (64.6%) met screening criteria.

For each student meeting screening criteria, parents were contacted to arrange a time for the diagnostic interview. We obtained informed consent and conducted a diagnostic interview with the parents of 76 students (80.0% of those who screened positively for ADHD). In each of these latter cases, the teacher completed the CAP a second time (CAP-2). Children were assigned to a diagnostic group or clinical control group on the basis of their scores on a multimethod assessment battery including the parent version of the DICA-R and the teacher-rated CAP-2. The ADHD Rating Scale–IV was not used to determine clinical group membership.

Children were categorized as having ADHD (any subtype) if they met criteria for any of the ADHD subtypes on the DICA-R and were rated by teachers as greater than or equal to the 93rd percentile on the Inattention and/or Overactivity subscale of the CAP-2. Using these criteria, 52 children were classified as having ADHD. Subtype membership was determined by the DICA-R; 29 students were diagnosed with ADHD/I, 0 with ADHD/HI, and 23 with ADHD/COM. In the sample, 76 students, including the 52 children not meeting initial screening criteria on the CAP, did not meet criteria for ADHD and were assigned to the control group. An additional 19 students met screening criteria through the use of the CAP, but we were not able to arrange a diagnostic interview with their parents.

Predictive Validity of the Inattention Subscale

Table 4.7 presents the results of logistic regression analyses used to evaluate the ability of the Inattention subscale of the ADHD Rating Scale–IV to differentiate children with ADHD/I from those in the control group. Both teacher and parent ratings, when entered separately, were predictive of membership in the ADHD/I group versus the control

TABLE 4.7. Results of Logistic Regression Analyses When Using the Inattention Subscale: School-Based Study

Comparison	χ^2	p	R	Prediction
ADHD/I versus control group				
Teacher ratings	15.65	.0001	.32	75%
Parent ratings	11.52	.001	.27	76%
ADHD/COM versus control group				
Teacher ratings	18.15	.0001	.36	78%
Parent ratings	20.30	.0001	.36	80%

group. The association between teacher ratings of Inattention and diagnostic status was low to moderate ($R = .32$), as was the association between parent ratings of Inattention and diagnostic status ($R = .27$). In a forward stepwise logistic regression analysis, teacher ratings entered the equation first. The addition of parent ratings resulted in a significant improvement of the logistic model ($\chi^2(1) = 7.90$, $p < .01$). The combination of teacher and parent ratings in the model correctly classified 78% of the cases.

Next, logistic regression analyses were used to evaluate the ability of the Inattention subscale to differentiate children with ADHD/COM from those in the control group (see Table 4.7). Both teacher ratings and parent ratings, when entered separately, were predictive of membership in the ADHD/COM group versus the control group. The association between teacher ratings of Inattention and diagnostic status was low to moderate ($R = .36$), as was the association between parent ratings of Inattention and diagnostic status ($R = .36$). In a forward stepwise logistic regression analysis, teacher ratings entered the equation first; the addition of parent ratings resulted in a significant improvement of the logistic model ($\chi^2(1) = 12.29$, $p < .001$). The combination of teacher and parent ratings in the model correctly classified 83% of the cases.

Predictive Validity of the Hyperactivity–Impulsivity Subscale

Logistic regression analyses were used to evaluate the ability of the Hyperactivity–Impulsivity subscale to differentiate children with ADHD/COM from those in the control group (see Table 4.8). Both teacher ratings and parent ratings, when entered separately, were able to predict membership in the ADHD/COM group versus the control group. The association between teacher ratings of Hyperactivity–Impulsivity and diagnostic status was low ($R = .26$), but the association between parent ratings of Hyperactivity–Impulsivity and diagnostic status was moderate ($R = .40$). In a forward stepwise logistic regression analysis, parent ratings entered the equation first. The addition of teacher ratings resulted in significant improvement of the logistic model

TABLE 4.8. Results of Logistic Regression Analyses When Using the Hyperactivity–Impulsivity Subscale: School-Based Study

Comparison	χ^2	p	R	Prediction
ADHD/COM versus control group				
Teacher ratings	9.88	.01	.26	78%
Parent ratings	22.51	.0001	.40	82%
ADHD/COM versus ADHD/I				
Teacher ratings	2.66	n.s.	.08	62%
Parent ratings	17.46	.0001	.39	79%

($\chi^2(1)$ = 6.04, p < .05). The combination of teacher and parent ratings in the model correctly classified 83% of the cases.

Next, logistic regression analyses were used to evaluate the ability of the Hyperactivity–Impulsivity subscale to differentiate children with ADHD/COM from those with ADHD/I (see Table 4.8). When teacher ratings were entered alone in the analysis, the resultant model was not able to differentiate children with ADHD/COM from those with ADHD/I at a statistically significant level. However, parent ratings, when entered alone, were able to differentiate ADHD/COM from ADHD/I and correctly classified 79% of the cases. The association between parent ratings of Hyperactivity–Impulsivity and diagnostic status was moderate (R = .39). In a forward stepwise logistic regression analysis, parent ratings only entered the equation first; the addition of teacher ratings did not result in a significant improvement of the logistic model.

Conclusions

The results of the school-based study indicated that the Inattention and Hyperactivity–Impulsivity subscales of the ADHD Rating Scale–IV were successful in predicting group membership in the ADHD/COM and ADHD/I groups. Logistic regression analyses revealed that the Inattention subscale was accurate in differentiating children with ADHD/I and ADHD/COM from the control group. Moreover, logistic regression analyses showed that the Hyperactivity–Impulsivity subscale successfully differentiated children with ADHD/COM from controls, as well as children with ADHD/COM from those with ADHD/I. The pattern of results differed somewhat, depending on whether the Inattention subscale or the Hyperactivity–Impulsivity subscale was being used for prediction. When predictions were based on the Inattention subscale, both teachers and parents made a significant and essentially equal contribution to the prediction of diagnostic status. This finding was demonstrated in the prediction of children with ADHD/I, as well as in the prediction of those with ADHD/COM. Even though teacher ratings entered the equation first in a forward stepwise analysis, parent ratings made an additional significant contribution to the prediction of diagnostic status.

In making predictions based on ratings on the Hyperactivity–Impulsivity subscale, parent ratings in general were more accurate than teacher ratings. Both teacher and parent ratings of Hyperactivity–Impulsivity made a significant contribution to the prediction of children with ADHD/COM versus those in the control group, but parent ratings clearly made a stronger contribution to prediction. Further, parent ratings, but not teacher ratings, of Hyperactivity–Impulsivity were successful in differentiating between the two subtypes of ADHD.

Summary and Conclusions

Our analyses indicate that the Home and School Versions of the ADHD Rating Scale–IV have adequate psychometric properties for use as screening, diagnostic and treatment outcome measures. Subscales on both versions of the rating scale were found to have high levels of internal consistency and test–retest reliability. Further, subscale scores were found to correlate significantly with questionnaires commonly used in the assessment of ADHD (i.e., the Conners Parent and Teacher Rating Scales). Teacher ratings of ADHD symptoms were found to correlate significantly with classroom behavioral observations and children's academic performance. Parent ratings were less likely to correlate with classroom behavioral and academic measures, presumably because parents were rating behavior in a different environment (i.e., the home). Parent and teacher ratings on the ADHD Rating Scale–IV were also demonstrated to discriminate between children representing different ADHD subtypes, as well as between children with ADHD and clinic-referred children who did not have ADHD. Finally, the combination of parent and teacher ratings was found to predict diagnosis of ADHD in the context of both clinic-based and school-based assessments. When used as part of a comprehensive assessment battery that includes diagnostic interviews, behavior observations, and related measures, the ADHD Rating Scale–IV can provide reliable and valid data regarding the frequency of ADHD symptoms.

CHAPTER 5

Interpretation and Use
of the Scales for Diagnostic
and Screening Purposes

In selecting a rating scale for assessing ADHD, it is not sufficient to know that the measure has acceptable psychometric properties. A clinician must also know how useful the measure is in diagnosing ADHD and screening out children who do not have this disorder. To evaluate the clinical utility of an instrument, it is important to examine its sensitivity and specificity as well as its positive predictive power (PPP) and negative predictive power (NPP). This chapter describes research we conducted to evaluate the clinical utility of the ADHD Rating Scale–IV in a parent-referred clinical setting and a teacher-referred, school setting. Case studies are presented to illustrate how to use this scale in clinical decision making.

Diagnosing ADHD

Sensitivity and PPP are very helpful statistics for determining the degree to which a measure is useful in diagnosing or "ruling in" a disorder. Sensitivity, as it pertains to the use of rating scales, refers to the probability that children known to have a disorder are rated at or above a particular cutoff score. For instance, if the sensitivity associated with a score at the 93rd percentile on a measure of Inattention is .90, this means that 90% of children known to have ADHD will score at or above this percentile. Sensitivity reflects the confidence one has in generalizing from a disorder to a behavior or score, which is a deductive process. In contrast, PPP refers to the probability that a child has a disorder, given the presence of a score at or above a designated cutoff point on a diagnostic measure. For instance, if the PPP associated with a score at the 93rd percentile on a measure of Inattention is .90, this means that 90% of children scoring at or above this cutoff point have ADHD. Thus, PPP represents the confidence a clinician can have in generalizing from a score to a disorder, which is the inductive process typically used in the clinical decision-making process.

Screening for ADHD

Specificity and NPP are helpful in determining the degree to which a measure is useful in screening to rule out a disorder. Specificity refers to the probability that children who do not have a certain disorder are rated below a particular cutoff score. For instance, if the specificity associated with a score at the 85th percentile on a measure of Inattention is .90, this means that 90% of children who do not have ADHD will score below this percentile. Like sensitivity, specificity reflects the confidence one has in generalizing from a disorder, to a behavior or score. In contrast, NPP refers to the probability that a child does not have a disorder given a score below a designated cutoff point on a diagnostic measure. For instance, if the NPP associated with a score at the 85th percentile on a measure of Inattention is .90, this means that 90% of children scoring below this cutoff score do not have ADHD. Like PPP, NPP represents the confidence a clinician can have in generalizing from a behavior or score to a disorder.

Several researchers have argued that in evaluating the clinical utility of a measure, PPP and NPP are more important than sensitivity and specificity (Chen, Faraone, Biederman, & Tsuang, 1994; Laurent, Landau, & Stark, 1993). In fact, both sets of constructs are important to consider in determining the utility of a measure and the optimal choice of cutoff scores, as will be illustrated later in this chapter.

Selecting the Optimal Cutoff Score

The choice of an optimal cutoff score on a scale varies, depending on the purpose of an assessment. If an examiner is performing a screening of ADHD in the general population of children, selection of a cutoff score that is highly accurate in predicting the absence of ADHD (NPP), as well as one that is able to detect a relatively high percentage of children that do not have ADHD (specificity), is very important. For screening, it is generally preferable to err on the side of being unduly *inclusive* of children with ADHD, as opposed to unduly exclusive of these youngsters, knowing that a more comprehensive evaluation conducted at at later time will provide more conclusive diagnostic information. However, when an examiner performs a diagnostic assessment, selection of a cutoff score that is highly accurate in predicting the presence of ADHD (PPP), as well as one that is able to detect a relatively high percentage of children known to have ADHD (sensitivity), is critical. For the purposes of diagnostic assessment, it is preferable to err on the side of being unduly *exclusive*. Given that the diagnosis of ADHD often has implications for medication use and school programming, it is important for the examiner to be quite certain of an accurate diagnosis and to identify few false positives.

Research on the Clinical Utility of the ADHD Rating Scale–IV

We conducted two studies, a clinic-based and a school-based study, to evaluate the clinical utility of the ADHD Rating Scale–IV (Power, Andrews, et al., in press; Power, Doherty, et al., 1998). The methodology for these studies is described in Chapter 4 in the sections on discriminant and predictive validity. For both the clinic-based sample and school-based sample, symptom utility estimates (sensitivity, specificity, PPP, and NPP) were used to determine optimal cutoff scores on the Inattention subscale of the ADHD Rating Scale–IV for differentiating (1) children with ADHD/I from a clinical control group without any subtype of ADHD and (2) children with ADHD/COM from clinical controls. Symptom utility estimates were also used to determine the optimal cutoff scores on the Hyperactivity–Impulsivity subscale for differentiating (1) children with ADHD/COM from clinical controls and (2) children with ADHD/I from those with ADHD/COM.

A problem with using PPP and NPP is that these statistics are highly sensitive to base rates of symptoms (cutoffs) and diagnoses in a sample (Verhulst & Koot, 1992). Thus, to make comparisons about the clinical utility of one cutoff score versus another, each of which may have a different base rate in the sample, it is necessary to employ a kappa statistic that corrects for the number of accurate predictions based on chance alone. Formulas for the kappa statistics used in our study to correct PPP (cPPP) and NPP (cNPP) were utilized in the DSM-IV field trials and are reported in Frick et al. (1994).

Prediction in a Clinic-Based Setting

Clinical Utility of the Inattention Subscale in a Clinic Setting

Children in the age range from 6 to 14 years participated in the clinic-based study. Symptom utility estimates associated with a series of possible cutoff scores on the Inattention subscale of the ADHD Rating Scale–IV, as rated by teachers and parents separately, are provided in Table 5.1. This table indicates base rates, sensitivity, specificity, PPP, cPPP, NPP, and cNPP statistics associated with each cutoff score (80th, 85th, 90th, 93rd, and 98th percentiles) investigated in the clinic-based study described in Chapter 4. Table 5.1 presents data regarding the ability of the Inattention subscale, as rated by teachers and parents, to differentiate children with ADHD/I from controls, as well as to differentiate children with ADHD/COM from the control group. The strategy for determining optimal thresholds was to identify the cutoff score associated with the highest level of accurate prediction (cPPP or cNPP) that resulted in a reasonable level of sensitivity or specificity. For purposes of this study, a cutoff score was considered clinically useful if cPPP or cNPP was greater than or equal to .65 and sensitivity or specificity was approximately .50 or greater.

Prediction Based on a Single Informant

The optimal cutoff score for differentiating children with ADHD/I from controls, using teacher ratings on the Inattention subscale, was the 98th percentile, but this

TABLE 5.1. Symptom Utility Estimates Associated with Cutoff Scores on the Inattention Subscale: Clinic-Based Study

Cutoff score	Base rate	Sensitivity	Specificity	PPP (cPPP)	NPP (cNPP)
Differentiating ADHD/I from controls—Teacher ratings					
≥ 98	.11	.20	.97	.85 (.73)	.59 (.10)
≥ 93	.37	.63	.86	.79 (.61)	.73 (.42)
≥ 90	.42	.67	.80	.74 (.52)	.74 (.43)
≥ 85	.54	.77	.66	.66 (.36)	.77 (.49)
≥ 80	.71	.90	.46	.59 (.23)	.84 (.66)
Differentiating ADHD/COM from controls—Teacher ratings					
≥ 98	.10	.20	.97	.83 (.71)	.63 (.11)
≥ 93	.38	.72	.86	.78 (.63)	.81 (.54)
≥ 90	.45	.80	.80	.74 (.56)	.85 (.64)
≥ 85	.55	.84	.66	.64 (.38)	.85 (.64)
≥ 80	.70	.92	.46	.55 (.22)	.89 (.73)
Differentiating ADHD/I from controls—Parent ratings					
≥ 98	.35	.47	.74	.61 (.27)	.62 (.17)
≥ 93	.66	.83	.49	.58 (.22)	.77 (.51)
≥ 90	.75	.93	.40	.57 (.20)	.88 (.73)
≥ 85	.77	.93	.37	.56 (.18)	.87 (.71)
≥ 80	.83	.93	.26	.52 (.11)	.82 (.61)
Differentiating ADHD/COM from controls—Parent ratings					
≥ 98	.27	.28	.74	.44 (.04)	.59 (.02)
≥ 93	.65	.84	.49	.54 (.21)	.81 (.54)
≥ 90	.73	.92	.40	.52 (.18)	.88 (.70)
≥ 85	.77	.96	.37	.52 (.18)	.93 (.83)
≥ 80	.85	1.00	.26	.49 (.13)	1.00 (1.00)

Note. Cutoff scores are percentile values. Base rate refers to the proportion of children in the clinical and control groups scoring at or above the specified cutoff score. PPP refers to positive predictive power and NPP refers to negative predictive power; cPPP and cNPP are kappa statistics used to correct PPP and NPP. From Power et al. (1998). Copyright 1998 by Plenum Publishing Corporation. Reprinted by permission.

was only marginally useful: 85% of the children scoring at or above this cutoff point had ADHD/I (cPPP = .73), but only 20% of children with ADHD/I scored at or above this level (sensitivity). The optimal cutoff score on the teacher-rated Inattention subscale for ruling out ADHD/I (80th percentile) was also marginally useful; 84% of children scoring below this cutoff point did not have ADHD/I (cNPP = .66), and 46% of children who did not have ADHD/I scored below this cutoff point (specificity).

Teacher ratings on the Inattention subscale were also marginally useful in predicting children who had ADHD/COM. The optimal cutoff score for ruling in ADHD/COM was the 98th percentile; the optimal cutoff for ruling out this subtype was the 80th percentile. As was the case when teacher ratings were used to differentiate ADHD/I from controls, cPPP and cNPP values were relatively high, but sensitivity and specificity values were quite low.

Parent ratings of Inattention were not useful in predicting or ruling in a diagnosis of ADHD/I or ADHD/COM. For ruling out ADHD/I, the 90th percentile was most useful: cNPP was relatively high (.73), but only 40% of children without ADHD/I scored below this cutoff point. For ruling out ADHD/COM, the 85th percentile had some utility: cNPP was high (.83), but only 37% of children without ADHD/COM scored below this cutoff point.

Prediction Based on Multiple Informants

Given that the results of logistic regression analyses demonstrated that the integration of teacher and parent ratings on the Inattention subscale was better than single-informant cutoff scores in predicting group membership (see Chapter 4), at least for children who met criteria for ADHD/I, symptom utility estimates for all possible combinations of parent and teacher ratings were computed. The combination cutoff scores for the Inattention subscale that had the highest level of utility for predicting ADHD/I and ADHD/COM are presented in Table 5.2. In general, the combination cutoff scores were better than the single scale thresholds in predicting or "ruling in" ADHD/I and ADHD/COM. For example, teacher ratings greater than or equal to the 90th percentile on the Inattention subscale were associated with a diagnosis of ADHD/I in 74% of cases (cPPP = .52). However, when teacher ratings greater than or equal to the 90th percentile were combined with parent ratings greater than or equal to the 93rd percentile, the rate of prediction improved to 85% (cPPP = .72) and sensitivity was still reasonably high (.57). The combination of parent and teacher ratings of Inattention was marginally useful in ruling out a diagnosis of ADHD/I; with teacher ratings below the 80th percentile and parent ratings below the 85th percentile, cNPP was moderate (.63) and specificity was .69.

In regard to differentiating children with ADHD/COM from controls, combination cutoff scores involving teacher ratings at or above the 90th percentile and parent ratings at or above the 93rd percentile, once again, constituted the optimal combination. For instance, this combination resulted in a high level of cPPP (.77) and a sensitivity of 76% in cases of children who met criteria for ADHD/COM. For ruling out ADHD/COM, teacher ratings below the 80th percentile and parent ratings below the 85th percentile had a high degree of utility: cNPP was .73, and 69% of children without ADHD/COM scored below these levels.

TABLE 5.2. Symptom Utility Estimates Associated with the Combination of Teacher (T) and Parent (P) Ratings on the Inattention Subscale: Clinic-Based Study

Cutoff score	Base rate	Sensitivity	Specificity	PPP (cPPP)	NPP (cNPP)
		Differentiating ADHD/I from controls			
T ≥ 80, P ≥ 80	.60	.83	.60	.64 (.33)	.81 (.58)
T ≥ 80, P ≥ 85	.55	.83	.69	.69 (.43)	.83 (.63)
T ≥ 80, P ≥ 90	.55	.83	.69	.69 (.43)	.83 (.63)
T ≥ 80, P ≥ 93	.49	.77	.74	.72 (.48)	.79 (.54)
T ≥ 80, P ≥ 98	.29	.43	.82	.68 (.41)	.63 (.20)
T ≥ 85, P ≥ 80	.46	.70	.74	.70 (.44)	.74 (.44)
T ≥ 85, P ≥ 85	.43	.70	.80	.75 (.54)	.76 (.47)
T ≥ 85, P ≥ 90	.43	.70	.80	.75 (.54)	.76 (.47)
T ≥ 85, P ≥ 93	.38	.67	.86	.80 (.63)	.75 (.46)
T ≥ 85, P ≥ 98	.23	.37	.89	.73 (.50)	.62 (.18)
T ≥ 90, P ≥ 80	.37	.60	.83	.75 (.54)	.71 (.37)
T ≥ 90, P ≥ 85	.35	.60	.86	.78 (.60)	.71 (.38)
T ≥ 90, P ≥ 90	.35	.60	.86	.78 (.60)	.71 (.38)
T ≥ 90, P ≥ 93	.31	.57	.91	.85 (.72)	.62 (.18)
T ≥ 90, P ≥ 98	.18	.33	.94	.83 (.69)	.62 (.18)
		Differentiating ADHD/COM from controls			
T ≥ 80, P ≥ 80	.62	.92	.60	.62 (.35)	.91 (.79)
T ≥ 80, P ≥ 85	.55	.88	.69	.67 (.43)	.89 (.73)
T ≥ 80, P ≥ 90	.53	.84	.69	.66 (.41)	.86 (.66)
T ≥ 80, P ≥ 93	.50	.84	.74	.70 (.49)	.87 (.68)
T ≥ 80, P ≥ 98	.22	.28	.83	.54 (.21)	.62 (.08)
T ≥ 85, P ≥ 80	.50	.84	.74	.70 (.49)	.87 (.68)
T ≥ 85, P ≥ 85	.47	.84	.80	.75 (.57)	.88 (.70)
T ≥ 85, P ≥ 90	.45	.80	.80	.74 (.56)	.85 (.64)
T ≥ 85, P ≥ 93	.42	.80	.86	.80 (.66)	.86 (.66)
T ≥ 85, P ≥ 98	.17	.24	.89	.60 (.31)	.62 (.09)
T ≥ 90, P ≥ 80	.43	.80	.83	.77 (.60)	.85 (.65)
T ≥ 90, P ≥ 85	.42	.80	.86	.80 (.66)	.86 (.66)
T ≥ 90, P ≥ 90	.40	.76	.86	.79 (.64)	.83 (.60)
T ≥ 90, P ≥ 93	.37	.76	.91	.86 (.77)	.84 (.62)
T ≥ 90, P ≥ 98	.13	.24	.94	.75 (.57)	.63 (.12)

Note. From Power et al. (1998). Copyright 1998 by Plenum Publishing Corporation. Reprinted by permission.

Clinical Utility of the Hyperactivity–Impulsivity Subscale in a Clinic Setting

Symptom utility estimates associated with a series of possible cutoff scores on the Hyperactivity–Impulsivity subscale of the ADHD Rating Scale-IV, as rated by teachers and parents separately, are provided in Table 5.3. This table presents data regarding the ability of the Hyperactivity–Impulsivity subscale to differentiate children with ADHD/COM from controls, as well as to differentiate children with ADHD/COM from those with ADHD/I.

TABLE 5.3. Symptom Utility Estimates Associated with Cutoff Scores on the Hyperactivity–Impulsivity Subscale: Clinic-Based Study

Cutoff score	Base rate	Sensitivity	Specificity	PPP (cPPP)	NPP (cNPP)
Differentiating ADHD/COM from controls—Teacher ratings					
≥ 98	.33	.48	.77	.60 (.31)	.68 (.22)
≥ 93	.47	.64	.66	.57 (.27)	.72 (.33)
≥ 90	.60	.88	.60	.61 (.33)	.88 (.70)
≥ 85	.67	.92	.51	.58 (.27)	.90 (.76)
≥ 80	.80	.96	.31	.50 (.14)	.92 (.80)
Differentiating ADHD/COM from ADHD/I—Teacher ratings					
≥ 98	.24	.48	.97	.92 (.86)	.69 (.32)
≥ 93	.35	.64	.90	.84 (.71)	.75 (.45)
≥ 90	.51	.88	.80	.79 (.61)	.89 (.76)
≥ 85	.60	.92	.67	.70 (.44)	.91 (.80)
≥ 80	.73	.96	.47	.60 (.27)	.93 (.85)
Differentiating ADHD/COM from controls—Parent ratings					
≥ 98	.45	.16	.63	.27 (−.34)	.47 (−.15)
≥ 93	.67	.53	.46	.46 (−.01)	.47 (−.01)
≥ 90	.68	.60	.43	.47 (.02)	.56 (.04)
≥ 85	.73	.67	.40	.49 (.05)	.58 (.10)
≥ 80	.78	.73	.26	.48 (.31)	.58 (.09)
Differentiating ADHD/COM from ADHD/I—Parent ratings					
≥ 98	.35	.56	.83	.74 (.52)	.69 (.33)
≥ 93	.67	.84	.47	.57 (.21)	.78 (.51)
≥ 90	.71	.84	.40	.54 (.15)	.75 (.45)
≥ 85	.78	.92	.33	.53 (.15)	.83 (.63)
≥ 80	.82	.92	.27	.51 (.10)	.80 (.56)

Note. From Power et al. (1998). Copyright 1998 by Plenum Publishing Corporation. Reprinted by permission

Prediction Based on a Single Informant

Teacher ratings of Hyperactivity–Impulsivity generally were not useful in predicting children who had ADHD/COM when this subtype was compared to controls; however, this scale was useful in ruling out a diagnosis of ADHD/COM. For instance, 90% of the children with teacher ratings below the 85th percentile did not have ADHD/COM (cNPP = .76), and 51% of the children who did not have ADHD/COM scored below this cutoff point (specificity). Parent ratings of Hyperactivity–Impulsivity were not useful in ruling in or ruling out ADHD/COM.

Teacher ratings on the Hyperactivity–Impulsivity subscale were much more useful in differentiating children with ADHD/COM from those with ADHD/I. The optimal cutoff score for predicting or ruling in ADHD/COM was the 98th percentile: 92% of children scoring at or above this level had ADHD/COM (cPPP = .86), and 48% of children with this subtype scored at or above the 98th percentile. The Hyperactivity–Impulsivity subscale was also useful in ruling out ADHD/COM when children with the two subtypes of ADHD were compared. For instance, teacher ratings below the 85th percentile resulted in a cNPP of .80 and a specificity of .67. Parent ratings of Hyperactivity–Impulsivity were not useful in ruling in or ruling out a diagnosis of ADHD/COM when children with the two subtypes of ADHD were compared and when children with ADHD/COM were compared to controls.

Prediction Based on Multiple Informants

Given that the results of logistic regression analyses demonstrated that the integration of teacher and parent ratings on the Hyperactivity–Impulsivity subscale was better than single-informant cutoff scores in predicting children who met criteria for ADHD/COM, at least when children with ADHD/COM were contrasted with the control group (see Chapter 4), symptom utility estimates for all possible combinations of parent and teacher ratings were computed. The combination cutoff scores with the most utility are presented in Table 5.4. As expected, based on the results of logistic regression analyses, the combination cutoff scores were better than teacher ratings alone in differentiating children with ADHD/COM from the control group, but not in differentiating children with ADHD/COM from those with ADHD/I. When the ADHD/COM group was compared with the control group, the optimal combination was teacher ratings at or above the 90th percentile and parent ratings at or above the 98th percentile; cPPP was moderate to high (.66) and 48% of children with ADHD/COM were identified. For ruling out ADHD/COM, both when the ADHD/COM group was compared with the control group and when the ADHD/COM group was compared with the ADHD/I group, the combination cutoff scores were not as accurate as teacher ratings alone.

Conclusions: Prediction in a Clinic Setting

Optimal cutoff scores for diagnosing and ruling out ADHD in our parent-referred, clinic-based sample are summarized in Table 5.5. The optimal approach for using the

TABLE 5.4. Symptom Utility Estimates Associated with the Combination of Teacher (T) and Parent (P) Ratings on the Hyperactivity--Impulsivity Subscale: Clinic-Based Study

Cutoff score	Base rate	Sensitivity	Specificity	PPP (cPPP)	NPP (cNPP)
		Differentiating ADHD/COM from controls			
T ≥ 80, P ≥ 80	.63	.88	.54	.58 (.28)	.86 (.67)
T ≥ 80, P ≥ 85	.62	.88	.57	.59 (.31)	.87 (.69)
T ≥ 80, P ≥ 90	.57	.80	.60	.59 (.29)	.81 (.54)
T ≥ 80, P ≥ 93	.55	.80	.63	.61 (.32)	.81 (.56)
T ≥ 80, P ≥ 98	.37	.56	.77	.64 (.38)	.71 (.31)
T ≥ 85, P ≥ 80	.53	.84	.69	.66 (.41)	.86 (.66)
T ≥ 85, P ≥ 85	.52	.84	.71	.68 (.45)	.86 (.67)
T ≥ 85, P ≥ 90	.47	.76	.74	.68 (.45)	.81 (.55)
T ≥ 85, P ≥ 93	.45	.76	.77	.70 (.49)	.82 (.56)
T ≥ 85, P ≥ 98	.28	.52	.88	.76 (.60)	.72 (.33)
T ≥ 90, P ≥ 80	.48	.80	.74	.68 (.47)	.84 (.61)
T ≥ 90, P ≥ 85	.47	.80	.77	.71 (.51)	.84 (.63)
T ≥ 90, P ≥ 90	.42	.72	.80	.72 (.52)	.80 (.52)
T ≥ 90, P ≥ 93	.40	.72	.83	.75 (.57)	.81 (.53)
T ≥ 90, P ≥ 98	.25	.48	.91	.80 (.66)	.71 (.31)
		Differentiating ADHD/COM from ADHD/I			
T ≥ 80, P ≥ 80	.67	.88	.50	.59 (.26)	.83 (.63)
T ≥ 80, P ≥ 85	.67	.88	.50	.59 (.26)	.83 (.63)
T ≥ 80, P ≥ 90	.64	.80	.50	.57 (.21)	.75 (.45)
T ≥ 80, P ≥ 93	.60	.80	.57	.61 (.28)	.77 (.50)
T ≥ 80, P ≥ 98	.35	.56	.83	.74 (.52)	.69 (.33)
T ≥ 85, P ≥ 80	.55	.84	.70	.70 (.45)	.84 (.65)
T ≥ 85, P ≥ 85	.55	.84	.70	.70 (.45)	.84 (.65)
T ≥ 85, P ≥ 90	.51	.76	.70	.68 (.41)	.78 (.51)
T ≥ 85, P ≥ 93	.47	.76	.77	.73 (.51)	.79 (.54)
T ≥ 85, P ≥ 98	.27	.52	.93	.87 (.76)	.70 (.34)
T ≥ 90, P ≥ 80	.45	.80	.83	.80 (.63)	.83 (.63)
T ≥ 90, P ≥ 85	.45	.80	.83	.80 (.63)	.83 (.63)
T ≥ 90, P ≥ 90	.42	.72	.83	.78 (.60)	.78 (.52)
T ≥ 90, P ≥ 93	.40	.72	.87	.82 (.67)	.79 (.53)
T ≥ 90, P ≥ 98	.24	.48	.97	.92 (.86)	.69 (.32)

Note. From Power et al. (1998). Copyright 1998 by Plenum Publishing Corporation. Reprinted by permission.

TABLE 5.5. Optimal Cutoff Scores for Diagnosing and Ruling Out ADHD: Clinic-Based Study

Diagnosing ADHD/I	Inattention subscale (teacher) ≥ 90th percentile
	Inattention subscale (parent) ≥ 93rd percentile
	Hyperactivity–Impulsivity subscale (teacher) ≤ 85th percentile
Ruling out ADHD/I	Inattention subscale (teacher) < 80th percentile
	Inattention subscale (parent) < 85th percentile
Diagnosing ADHD/COM	Inattention subscale (teacher) ≥ 90th percentile
	Inattention subscale (parent) ≥ 93rd percentile
	Hyperactivity–Impulsivity subscale (teacher) ≥ 98th percentile
Ruling out ADHD/COM	Inattention subscale (teacher) < 80th percentile
	Inattention subscale (parent) < 85th percentile
	Hyperactivity–Impulsivity subscale (teacher) < 85th percentile

Note. The informant is indicated in parentheses.

Inattention subscale to predict the presence of ADHD/I and ADHD/COM was one that combined teacher and parent ratings. The most useful combination appeared to be teacher ratings at or above the 90th percentile and parent ratings at or above the 93rd percentile. The optimal approach to using the Inattention subscale to rule out the presence of ADHD was also a multi-informant one: Teacher ratings less than the 80th percentile and parent ratings less than the 85th percentile had the most utility.

The Hyperactivity–Impulsivity subscale had limited utility in differentiating the ADHD/COM group from the control group. However, this scale was useful in differentiating the ADHD/COM group from the ADHD/I group. The optimal approach to ruling in ADHD/COM when ADHD/COM and ADHD/I were compared was a single-informant strategy using teacher ratings at or above the 98th percentile. The most useful approach to ruling out ADHD/COM when the two subtypes were compared also appeared to be a single-informant approach using teacher ratings below the 85th percentile.

Given that the Inattention subscale generally was more useful than the Hyperactivity–Impulsivity subscale in differentiating children with ADHD from those in the control group, a helpful strategy is to decide first whether a referred child has a disorder of inattention (either ADHD/I or ADHD/COM), using the Inattention subscale. The optimal cutoff scores reported in Table 5.5 should be helpful in making this determination. Next, if the clinician determines that the child has ADHD/I or ADHD/COM, the Hyperactivity–Impulsivity subscale can be very useful in identifying the most appropriate subtype, using the recommended cutoff scores delineated in Table 5.5.

It is important to note that 24% of children who actually had ADHD/COM and 43% of children who had ADHD/I were missed when the optimal cutoff scores on the Inattention subscale determined in this study were used. Moreover, in 52% of the cases, the Hyperactivity–Impulsivity subscale failed to sort out who had ADHD/COM versus ADHD/I when the optimal cutoff score on the teacher rating scale was used. Thus, clinicians need to be cautious in the use of teacher and parent ratings of DSM-IV symptoms in determining whether ADHD exists and what subtype is most descriptive of the child. At this point, a strategy that incorporates teacher and parent ratings on the ADHD Rating Scale–IV along with information derived from other measures (e.g., diagnostic interviews and behavioral observations) is recommended in the diagnostic assessment of ADHD.

Given that there were so few children with ADHD/HI in this sample, it was not possible to investigate the ability of the Hyperactivity–Impulsivity subscale to differentiate children with ADHD/HI from controls. A useful guideline at this point is to consider the possibility of a diagnosis of ADHD/HI when the Inattentive or Combined subtype of ADHD can be ruled out (i.e., teacher ratings on the Inattention subscale are less than the 80th percentile and parent ratings on this scale are less than the 85th percentile), but a Hyperactive–Impulsive subtype of ADHD cannot be ruled out (i.e., teacher ratings on the Hyperactivity–Impulsivity subscale are greater than or equal to the 85th percentile).

The results of this study are generalizable to clinic-based settings serving children in the age range from 6 to 14 years. The findings may be less applicable in other settings, including school-based programs and clinics serving preschool children or older adolescents. Use of the kappa correction statistics for PPP and NPP mitigates variations in predictability across settings that have differential base rates for symptoms and disorders (Chen et al., 1994; Frick et al., 1994). However, fundamental differences between settings in regard to referral agent (parent versus teacher) and type of functional impairment may result in cross-situational inconsistencies in prediction that are not entirely corrected by kappa statistics. In using the ADHD Rating Scale–IV to make clinical decisions regarding children referred by teachers in a school setting, the guidelines described in the following sections should be more accurate and useful. Furthermore, clinicians need to be cautious about using the recommended cutoff scores in Table 5.5 with children who belong to ethnic minority groups (see Chapter 3).

Prediction in a School-Based Setting

Clinical Utility of the Inattention Subscale in a School Setting

Participants in the teacher-referred, school-based study included children in kindergarten through grade 8. Symptom utility estimates, including base rate, sensitivity, specificity, PPP, cPPP, NPP, and cNPP, for several possible cutoff scores (80th, 85th, 90th, 93rd, and 98th percentiles) on the Inattention subscale, as rated by teachers and parents, were computed. These are presented in Table 5.6. The strategy for determining

TABLE 5.6. Symptom Utility Estimates Associated with Cutoff Scores on the Inattention Subscale: School-Based Study

Cutoff score	Base rate	Sensitivity	Specificity	PPP (cPPP)	NPP (cNPP)
Differentiating ADHD/I from controls—Teacher ratings					
≥ 98	.06	.14	.97	.67 (.54)	.75 (.09)
≥ 93	.16	.34	.91	.59 (.43)	.78 (.22)
≥ 90	.21	.45	.88	.59 (.43)	.81 (.30)
≥ 85	.30	.59	.82	.55 (.38)	.84 (.41)
≥ 80	.42	.86	.75	.57 (.40)	.93 (.76)
Differentiating ADHD/COM from controls—Teacher ratings					
≥ 98	.03	.04	.97	.33 (.13)	.77 (.01)
≥ 93	.15	.35	.91	.53 (.39)	.82 (.23)
≥ 90	.22	.57	.88	.59 (.47)	.87 (.44)
≥ 85	.31	.74	.82	.55 (.41)	.91 (.62)
≥ 80	.37	.78	.75	.49 (.33)	.92 (.65)
Differentiating ADHD/I from controls—Parent ratings					
≥ 98	.11	.28	.95	.67 (.54)	.77 (.18)
≥ 93	.29	.48	.79	.47 (.26)	.80 (.28)
≥ 90	.36	.59	.72	.45 (.24)	.82 (.35)
≥ 85	.55	.76	.53	.38 (.14)	.85 (.46)
≥ 80	.67	.90	.41	.36 (.12)	.91 (.68)
Differentiating ADHD/COM from controls—Parent ratings					
≥ 98	.11	.30	.95	.64 (.53)	.82 (.22)
≥ 93	.30	.61	.79	.47 (.31)	.87 (.44)
≥ 90	.38	.74	.72	.45 (.28)	.90 (.58)
≥ 85	.57	.91	.53	.37 (.18)	.95 (.80)
≥ 80	.66	.96	.41	.32 (.12)	.97 (.87)

optimal thresholds was to identify the cutoff score associated with the highest level of accurate prediction (cPPP or cNPP) that resulted in a reasonable level of sensitivity or specificity. For purposes of this study, a cutoff score was considered clinically useful if cPPP or cNPP was greater than or equal to .65 and sensitivity or specificity was approximately .50 or greater.

Prediction Based on a Single Informant

The results indicated that single informant ratings of Inattention at the thresholds examined in this study were not useful in predicting the presence of ADHD/I or

ADHD/COM. When the Inattention subscale was used to differentiate children with ADHD/I and ADHD/COM from those in the control group, cPPP statistics were well below an acceptable level at each of the cutoff scores examined, as rated by both teachers and parents, even though in some cases sensitivity values were high. For example, although parent ratings greater than or equal to the 85th percentile were useful in detecting 91% of the children who met the criteria for ADHD/COM versus the control group (sensitivity), only 37% of children who scored at or above this cutoff score were diagnosed with ADHD/I (PPP), resulting in a cPPP value of .18.

In contrast, parent and teacher ratings on the Inattention subscale generally were highly useful in ruling out diagnoses. Teacher ratings below the 80th percentile were able to rule out ADHD/I in 93% of the cases (cNPP = .76), and 75% of the cases without a diagnosis of ADHD fell below this cutoff score (specificity). The same cutoff score was also able to rule out ADHD/COM in 92% of the cases (cNPP = .65) with a specificity of .75. Parent ratings on the Inattention subscale were also useful in ruling out ADHD/I and ADHD/COM, but they appeared somewhat less useful than teacher ratings. Parent ratings below the 80th percentile were able to rule out ADHD/I in 91% of the cases (cNPP = .68), but the specificity associated with this cutoff score was only .41. Similarly, this cutoff score was able to rule out ADHD/COM in 97% of the cases (cNPP = .87) with a specificity of .41.

Prediction Based on Multiple Informants

Given the results of logistic regression analyses demonstrating that the combination of teacher and parent ratings on the Inattention subscale was more effective than a single-informant approach in differentiating children with ADHD/I and ADHD/COM from those in the control group (see Chapter 4), symptom utility estimates for all possible combinations of teacher and parent ratings were computed. In general, the combination cutoff scores were better than the single-informant thresholds in predicting or ruling in ADHD/I and ADHD/COM. The combination cutoff scores that had the highest level of utility in predicting subtype membership are presented in Table 5.7. Combinations involving teacher ratings greater than or equal to the 93rd percentile were not included, because these were associated with very low rates of sensitivity and cNPP. For the prediction of both ADHD/I and ADHD/COM, the optimal combination was a teacher rating at or above the 90th percentile and a parent rating at or above the 80th percentile. In predicting a diagnosis of ADHD/I, this combination of scores was associated with a cPPP of .65, but a sensitivity of only .41. For predicting a diagnosis of ADHD/COM, this combination yielded a cPPP value of .67 and a sensitivity of .52. Thus, the optimal combination of cutoff values had a moderately high rate of prediction but failed to predict about 50% of the children who had ADHD/I or ADHD/COM. Combining teacher and parent ratings on the Inattention subscale was not as useful as a single informant approach in ruling out diagnoses of ADHD.

TABLE 5.7. Symptom Utility Estimates Associated with the Combination of Teacher (T) and Parent (P) Ratings on the Inattention Subscale: School-Based Study

Cutoff score	Base rate	Sensitivity	Specificity	PPP (cPPP)	NPP (cNPP)
		Differentiating ADHD/I from controls			
T ≥ 80, P ≥ 80	.32	.76	.84	.65 (.51)	.90 (.64)
T ≥ 80, P ≥ 85	.27	.66	.88	.68 (.56)	.87 (.53)
T ≥ 80, P ≥ 90	.20	.52	.92	.71 (.61)	.83 (.40)
T ≥ 80, P ≥ 93	.17	.45	.93	.72 (.62)	.82 (.33)
T ≥ 80, P ≥ 98	.09	.24	.97	.78 (.69)	.77 (.17)
T ≥ 85, P ≥ 80	.21	.70	.91	.68 (.56)	.83 (.39)
T ≥ 85, P ≥ 85	.18	.70	.92	.68 (.56)	.81 (.33)
T ≥ 85, P ≥ 90	.13	.61	.93	.64 (.51)	.78 (.20)
T ≥ 85, P ≥ 93	.12	.48	.95	.69 (.57)	.78 (.21)
T ≥ 85, P ≥ 98	.06	.22	.99	.83 (.77)	.76 (.12)
T ≥ 90, P ≥ 80	.15	.41	.95	.75 (.65)	.81 (.31)
T ≥ 90, P ≥ 85	.13	.34	.95	.71 (.61)	.79 (.24)
T ≥ 90, P ≥ 90	.10	.24	.95	.64 (.50)	.77 (.15)
T ≥ 90, P ≥ 93	.10	.24	.95	.64 (.50)	.77 (.15)
T ≥ 90, P ≥ 98	.05	.14	.99	.80 (.72)	.75 (.09)
		Differentiating ADHD/COM from controls			
T ≥ 80, P ≥ 80	.29	.74	.84	.59 (.46)	.91 (.63)
T ≥ 80, P ≥ 85	.25	.70	.88	.64 (.53)	.91 (.59)
T ≥ 80, P ≥ 90	.20	.61	.92	.70 (.61)	.89 (.51)
T ≥ 80, P ≥ 93	.16	.48	.93	.69 (.59)	.86 (.38)
T ≥ 80, P ≥ 98	.07	.22	.97	.71 (.63)	.80 (.16)
T ≥ 85, P ≥ 80	.23	.70	.91	.70 (.60)	.91 (.60)
T ≥ 85, P ≥ 85	.22	.70	.92	.73 (.64)	.91 (.61)
T ≥ 85, P ≥ 90	.18	.61	.93	.74 (.66)	.89 (.52)
T ≥ 85, P ≥ 93	.15	.48	.95	.73 (.65)	.86 (.39)
T ≥ 85, P ≥ 98	.06	.22	.99	.83 (.78)	.81 (.17)
T ≥ 90, P ≥ 80	.16	.52	.95	.75 (.67)	.87 (.43)
T ≥ 90, P ≥ 85	.16	.52	.95	.75 (.67)	.87 (.43)
T ≥ 90, P ≥ 90	.15	.48	.95	.73 (.65)	.86 (.39)
T ≥ 90, P ≥ 93	.13	.39	.95	.69 (.60)	.84 (.30)
T ≥ 90, P ≥ 98	.06	.22	.99	.83 (.78)	.81 (.17)

Note. From Power et al. (in press). Copyright by the American Psychological Association. Reprinted by permission.

Clinical Utility of the Hyperactivity–Impulsivity Subscale in a School Setting

Prediction Based on a Single Informant

Symptom utility estimates for several possible cutoff scores (80th, 85th, 90th, 93rd, and 98th percentiles) on the Hyperactivity–Impulsivity subscale of the ADHD Rating Scale-IV, as rated by teachers and parents, were computed and are presented in Table 5.8. Teacher ratings of Hyperactivity–Impulsivity generally were not useful in predicting or ruling in diagnostic group membership. Parent ratings at or above the 98th percentile on the Hyperactivity–Impulsivity subscale were able to differentiate children with ADHD/COM from the control group at a moderate to high level (cPPP = .67), but only

TABLE 5.8. Symptom Utility Estimates Associated with Cutoff Scores on the Hyperactivity–Impulsivity Subscale: School-Based Study

Cutoff score	Base rate	Sensitivity	Specificity	PPP (cPPP)	NPP (cNPP)
Differentiating ADHD/COM from controls–Teacher ratings					
≥ 98	.04	.09	.97	.50 (.35)	.78 (.05)
≥ 93	.09	.22	.95	.56 (.42)	.80 (.14)
≥ 90	.12	.30	.93	.58 (.46)	.82 (.21)
≥ 85	.20	.48	.88	.55 (.41)	.85 (.35)
≥ 80	.28	.61	.82	.50 (.35)	.87 (.45)
Differentiating ADHD/COM from ADHD/I–Teacher ratings					
≥ 98	.06	.09	.97	.67 (.40)	.57 (.03)
≥ 93	.17	.22	.86	.56 (.20)	.58 (.05)
≥ 90	.21	.30	.86	.64 (.35)	.61 (.12)
≥ 85	.33	.48	.79	.65 (.37)	.66 (.22)
≥ 80	.46	.61	.66	.58 (.25)	.68 (.27)
Differentiating ADHD/COM from controls–Parent ratings					
≥ 98	.08	.26	.97	.75 (.67)	.81 (.20)
≥ 93	.21	.52	.88	.57 (.44)	.86 (.39)
≥ 90	.30	.65	.80	.50 (.35)	.88 (.50)
≥ 85	.39	.78	.72	.46 (.30)	.92 (.64)
≥ 80	.48	.87	.63	.42 (.24)	.94 (.75)
Differentiating ADHD/COM from ADHD/I–Parent ratings					
≥ 98	.15	.26	.93	.75 (.55)	.61 (.13)
≥ 93	.29	.52	.90	.80 (.64)	.70 (.33)
≥ 90	.35	.65	.90	.83 (.70)	.76 (.47)
≥ 85	.50	.78	.72	.69 (.45)	.81 (.57)
≥ 80	.60	.87	.62	.65 (.36)	.86 (.68)

26% of children with ADHD/COM scored above this cutoff score on the ADHD Rating Scale–IV (sensitivity). However, it should be noted that parent ratings at or above the 90th percentile were quite useful in predicting children with ADHD/COM as opposed to ADHD/I; with the use of this cutoff score cPPP was .70 and sensitivity was .65.

Parent ratings on the Hyperactivity–Impulsivity subscale were useful in ruling out diagnostic group membership, but teacher ratings were not. Parent ratings below the 80th percentile were able to rule out ADHD/COM in 94% of the cases (cNPP = .75) with a specificity of .63. Parent ratings below this cutoff score were also able to rule out the Combined subtype, when children with ADHD/I were compared with those with ADHD/COM, in 86% of the cases (cNPP = .68) with a specificity of .62.

Prediction Based on Multiple Informants

Given the results of logistic regression analyses demonstrating that the combination of teacher and parent ratings on the Hyperactivity–Impulsivity subscale was more effective than a single informant approach in differentiating children with ADHD/COM from those in the control group, but not differentiating children with ADHD/COM from those with ADHD/I (see Chapter 4), symptom utility estimates for all possible combinations of teacher and parent ratings were computed. In general, the combination cutoff scores were better than the single informant thresholds in predicting or ruling in subtype membership. The combination cutoff scores that had the highest level of utility in predicting subtype membership are presented in Table 5.9. Combinations involving teacher ratings greater than or equal to the 93rd percentile were not included, because these were associated with very low rates of sensitivity and cNPP. For the prediction of ADHD/COM, the optimal combination was a teacher rating at or above the 80th percentile and a parent rating at or above the 85th percentile. In predicting children with ADHD/COM as compared with the control group, this combination of scores was associated with a cPPP of .74, and a sensitivity of .52. For predicting children with ADHD/COM as compared with those with ADHD/I, this combination yielded a cPPP value of .86 and a sensitivity of .52. Thus, the optimal combination of cutoff values had a high rate of prediction but failed to predict about 50% of the children who had ADHD/COM. Combining teacher and parent ratings on the Hyperactivity–Impulsivity subscale was not as useful as a single-informant approach in ruling out diagnoses of ADHD.

Conclusions: Prediction in a School Setting

Optimal cutoff scores for diagnosing and ruling out ADHD in our teacher-referred, school-based sample are summarized in Table 5.10. The results pointed to the conclusion that in a school-based sample of children referred by teachers, a single-informant approach is best for ruling out ADHD, whereas a combined approach is more useful in ruling this disorder in. The results further suggested that teacher and parent reports of ADHD symptoms, as assessed by the ADHD Rating Scale–IV, may be more useful in ruling out ADHD than ruling it in.

TABLE 5.9. Symptom Utility Estimates Associated with the Combination of Teacher (T) and Parent (P) Ratings on the Hyperactivity--Impulsivity Subscale: School-Based Study

Cutoff score	Base rate	Sensitivity	Specificity	PPP (cPPP)	NPP (cNPP)
		Differentiating ADHD/COM from controls			
T ≥ 80, P ≥ 80	.16	.52	.95	.75 (.67)	.87 (.43)
T ≥ 80, P ≥ 85	.15	.52	.96	.80 (.74)	.87 (.44)
T ≥ 80, P ≥ 90	.12	.39	.96	.75 (.67)	.84 (.31)
T ≥ 80, P ≥ 93	.09	30	.97	.78 (.71)	.82 (.23)
T ≥ 80, P ≥ 98	.03	.13	1.00	1.00 (1.00)	.79 (.10)
T ≥ 85, P ≥ 80	.13	.43	.96	.77 (.70)	.85 (.35)
T ≥ 85, P ≥ 85	.12	.43	.97	.83 (.78)	.85 (.36)
T ≥ 85, P ≥ 90	.09	.30	.97	.78 (.71)	.82 (.23)
T ≥ 85, P ≥ 93	.07	.22	.97	.71 (.63)	.80 (.16)
T ≥ 85, P ≥ 98	.02	.09	1.00	1.00 (1.00)	.78 (.07)
T ≥ 90, P ≥ 80	.08	.26	.97	.75 (.67)	.81 (.20)
T ≥ 90, P ≥ 85	.08	.26	.97	.75 (.67)	.81 (.20)
T ≥ 90, P ≥ 90	.06	.17	.97	.67 (.57)	.80 (.12)
T ≥ 90, P ≥ 93	.05	.13	.97	.60 (.48)	.79 (.08)
T ≥ 90, P ≥ 98	.02	.09	1.00	1.00 (1.00)	.78 (.07)
		Differentiating ADHD/COM from ADHD/I			
T ≥ 80, P ≥ 80	.27	.52	.93	.86 (.74)	.71 (.35)
T ≥ 80, P ≥ 85	.25	.52	.97	.92 (.86)	.72 (.36)
T ≥ 80, P ≥ 90	.19	.39	.97	.90 (.82)	.67 (.25)
T ≥ 80, P ≥ 93	.15	.30	.97	.88 (.78)	.64 (.18)
T ≥ 80, P ≥ 98	.08	.13	.97	.75 (.55)	.58 (.06)
T ≥ 85, P ≥ 80	.21	.43	.97	.91 (.84)	.68 (.28)
T ≥ 85, P ≥ 85	.19	.43	1.00	1.00 (1.00)	.69(.30)
T ≥ 85, P ≥ 90	.13	.30	1.00	1.00 (1.00)	.64 (.20)
T ≥ 85, P ≥ 93	.10	.22	1.00	1.00 (1.00)	.62 (.13)
T ≥ 85, P ≥ 98	.04	.09	1.00	1.00 (1.00)	.58 (.05)
T ≥ 90, P ≥ 80	.12	.26	1.00	1.00 (1.00)	.63 (.16)
T ≥ 90, P ≥ 85	.12	.26	1.00	1.00 (1.00)	.63 (.16)
T ≥ 90, P ≥ 90	.08	.17	1.00	1.00 (1.00)	.60 (.11)
T ≥ 90, P ≥ 93	.06	.13	1.00	1.00 (1.00)	.59 (.08)
T ≥ 90, P ≥ 98	.04	.09	1.00	1.00 (1.00)	.58 (.05)

Note. From Power et al. (in press). Copyright 1998 by the American Psychological Association. Reprinted by permission.

TABLE 5.10. Optimal Cutoff Scores for Diagnosing and Ruling Out ADHD in the Teacher-Referred, School-Based Sample: School-Based Study

Diagnosing ADHD/I	Inattention subscale (teacher) $\geq$ 90th percentile
	Inattention subscale (parent) $\geq$ 80th percentile
	Hyperactivity–Impulsivity subscale (parent) $\leq$ 80th percentile
Ruling out ADHD/I	Inattention subscale (teacher) < 80th percentile
Diagnosing ADHD/COM	Inattention subscale (teacher) $\geq$ 90th percentile
	Inattention subscale (parent) $\geq$ 80th percentile
	Hyperactivity–Impulsivity subscale (teacher) $\geq$ 80th percentile
	Hyperactivity–Impulsivity subscale (parent) $\geq$ 85th percentile
Ruling out ADHD/COM	Inattention subscale (teacher) < 80th percentile
	Hyperactivity–Impulsivity subscale (parent) < 80th percentile

Note. The informant is indicated in parentheses.

The Inattention subscale, rated by either teachers or parents, was quite successful in ruling out children with ADHD/I and ADHD/COM, although teacher reports appeared somewhat more accurate and useful than parent reports. Ratings by teachers below the 80th percentile on the Inattention subscale were optimal in ruling out ADHD. The combined-informant approach was more successful in predicting the presence of ADHD than the single-informant approach. For example, teacher ratings on the Inattention subscale at or above the 90th percentile were accurate in predicting ADHD/COM 59% of the time (cPPP =.47). However, when teacher ratings at or above the 90th percentile were combined with parent ratings at or above the 80th percentile, the prediction rate increased to 75% (cPPP = .65). Although prediction was improved with the combined-informant approach, cPPP was only moderately high and sensitivity was relatively low.

The Hyperactivity–Impulsivity subscale rated by parents, but not by teachers, was useful in ruling out a diagnosis of ADHD/COM. Parent ratings at or below the 80th percentile resulted in a moderate to high level of predictive power (cNPP of .68 to .75) and were successful in ruling out ADHD/COM with a reasonable level of specificity (.62 to .63). For predicting or ruling in ADHD/COM, the combined informant approach using the Hyperactivity–Impulsivity subscale demonstrated superiority over a single-informant approach. For example, teacher ratings on the Hyperactivity–Impulsivity subscale at or above the 80th percentile were successful in differentiating between children in the ADHD/COM group and children in the control group 50% of the time (cPPP = .35). However, when teacher ratings at or above the 80th percentile were combined with parent ratings at or above the 85th percentile, the prediction rate increased to 80% (cPPP = .74). This combination produced a high prediction rate, but a relatively low sensitivity rate (.52).

The ADHD Rating Scale–IV appears to be most useful in a school setting as a screening measure to be included in a multigate assessment process. Teacher ratings of Inattention were more useful than parent ratings in ruling out a disorder involving inattention (ADHD/I and ADHD/COM); parent ratings of Hyperactivity–Impulsivity were more useful than teacher ratings in ruling out ADHD/COM. The results of this study generally do not support the practice of using teacher and parent ratings alone or in combination in making diagnostic decisions about the presence of ADHD. Even though using a combination of teacher and parent reports of ADHD symptoms yielded a more accurate prediction of the presence of ADHD than a single-informant approach, predictive power and sensitivity generally were not high when the combined method was used, particularly when the Inattention subscale was used to predict ADHD/I and ADHD/COM. A more sensible approach is to use teacher and parent ratings in conjunction with other methods, such as diagnostic interviews and direct observation procedures, in making diagnostic decisions about ADHD.

Given that there were no students in this sample who had ADHD/HI, it was not possible to evaluate the ability of the ADHD Rating Scale–IV to predict this subtype. A useful guideline at this point is to consider the possibility of a diagnosis of ADHD/HI when an Inattentive subtype of ADHD can be ruled out (i.e., teacher ratings on the Inattention subscale are less than the 80th percentile), but a Hyperactive-Impulsive subtype of ADHD cannot be ruled out (i.e., parent ratings on the Hyperactivity–Impulsivity subscale are greater than or equal to the 80th percentile).

The results of this study are generalizable to samples of children referred to school-based child evaluation and treatment teams for attention, learning, and behavior problems. The use of kappa correction statistics for PPP and NPP mitigates variations in predictability across settings that have different base rates for symptoms and disorders (Chen et al., 1994; Frick et al., 1994). Nonetheless, it is possible that differences between settings (e.g., psychiatric clinic versus school-based team) in regard to referral agent and primary areas of functional impairment may result in cross-situational differences that cannot be entirely corrected statistically. Additional research is needed to identify the optimal approach to using teacher and parent report data among samples of referred children that differ by setting, referral source, and primary areas of functional impairment. As indicated earlier in this chapter, clinicians must be careful about using recommended cutoff scores in making clinical decisions about children belonging to ethnic minority groups.

Case Examples

Darnell

Darnell was referred to a hospital-based clinic by his parents because of their concerns about his inattention and behavior problems. Darnell is an African-American student who lives in a poor, urban environment. Teacher ratings on the ADHD Rating Scale–IV indicated that he was at the 93rd percentile on the Inattention subscale and at the 93rd percentile on the Hyperactivity–Impulsivity subscale. His mother rated him on this measure at the 93rd percentile for Inattention and at the 90th percentile for Hyperactivity–Impulsivity. Given that ratings from teachers and parents on the Inattention subscale were above the optimal cutoff scores for predicting or ruling in ADHD/COM and ADHD/I in a parent-referred clinic setting (see Table 5.5), it is likely that Darnell meets the criteria for ADHD. However, given that Darnell is an African-American student, clinicians should interpret normative data and recommended cutoff scores cautiously (Reid et al., 1998). Further, because teacher ratings on the Hyperactivity–Impulsivity subscale were below the optimal cutoff score for predicting ADHD/COM (98th percentile), it is unclear from rating scale data whether a diagnosis of ADHD/COM or ADHD/I is more appropriate. The clinician should interview the parent and review school information carefully to determine whether problems with behavioral control are contributing to functional problems at home and/or in school, which would be useful in determining whether there is a sufficient level of hyperactivity–impulsivity to warrant a diagnosis of ADHD/COM versus ADHD/I.

Jennifer

Jennifer was referred by her teacher to the school's Instructional Support Team because of concerns related to attention, learning, and behavior problems. Jennifer is a Caucasian student living in a middle-class suburban neighborhood. Teacher ratings were at the 93rd percentile on the Inattention subscale and at the 50th percentile on the Hyperactivity–Impulsivity subscale. Parent ratings were at the 90th percentile on the Inattention subscale and at the 75th percentile on the Hyperactivity–Impulsivity subscale. Teacher and parent ratings on the Inattention subscale strongly suggested the presence of ADHD (see Table 5.10). Because parent and teacher ratings on the Hyperactivity–Impulsivity subscale were relatively low and within the range where ADHD/COM could be ruled out, the data strongly suggest the presence of ADHD/I. The clincian should review assessment findings to confirm this diagnosis.

Robert

Robert was referred to a community-based clinic by his parents because of their concern about his learning and behavior problems. Robert is a Caucasian child from a working-class neighborhood. Teacher ratings on the ADHD Rating Scale–IV indicated that he was at the 93rd percentile on the Inattention subscale and at the 90th percentile on the Hyperactivity–Impulsivity subscale. Parent ratings on this measure revealed percentile scores of 85 for Inattention and 85 for Hyperactivity–Impulsivity. Teacher ratings of Inattention were above the optimal cutoff score for diagnosing ADHD, but parent ratings were not (see Table 5.5). Further, teacher and parent ratings on the Hyperactivity–Impulsivity subscale were not below the thresholds for ruling out ADHD/COM or ADHD/I. In this case, the diagnosis is unclear. It is recommended that the clinician interview the parents, review school information, and conduct a direct observation of the child in school, if possible, to sort out diagnostic issues.

Maria

Maria was referred by her teacher to the school's Instructional Support Team because of concern about her attention and learning problems. Maria is a child of Latino background who lives in a rural setting. Teacher ratings on the ADHD Rating Scale–IV were at the 75th percentile for Inattention and at 75th percentile for Hyperactivity–Impulsivity. Parent ratings on the Inattention subscale were at the 50th percentile and at the 75th percentile for Hyperactivity–Impulsivity. Given that teacher and parent ratings on both the Inattention and Hyperactivity–Impulsivity subscales were below the cutoff scores for ruling out ADHD in a teacher-referred school sample (see Table 5.10), it is not likely that Maria meets the criteria for this disorder. However, before ruling out ADHD conclusively, the clinician should review the historical data presented by the family as well as school records.

Sharlene

Sharlene was referred by her teacher to the school's Instructional Support Team because of concerns related to attention, learning, and behavior problems. Sharlene is an African-American student living in an upper-middle-class neighborhood. Teacher ratings on the ADHD Rating Scale–IV were at the 93rd percentile on the Inattention subscale and at the 90th percentile on the Hyperactivity–Impulsivity subscale. Parent ratings were at the 90th percentile on the Inattention subscale and at the 80th percentile on the Hyperactivity–Impulsivity subscale. Teacher and parent ratings on the Inattention subscale strongly suggested the presence of ADHD (see Table 5.10); however, recommended cutoff scores should be interpreted cautiously with children who are African-American. Ratings on the Hyperactivity–Impulsivity subscale were inconclusive about subtype. Teacher ratings were above the recommended cutoff score for ruling in ADHD/COM, but parent ratings were below the optimal threshold. Additional information is needed to confirm the presence of ADHD and to clarify the child's subtype.

Charles

After conferring with his parents, his teacher referred Charles to the school's Mainstream Assistance Team because of concerns about problems in following directions and controlling his behavior, which were interfering with academic achievement and peer relationships. Teacher ratings on the ADHD Rating Scale–IV were above the 93rd percentile on both subscales. Parent ratings on this measure were above the 85th percentile on each subscale. In light of the guidelines presented in Table 5.10, the evidence strongly suggested the presence of ADHD/COM. Before sharing conclusions with the parents, the clinician should review clinical findings to confirm the diagnosis.

CHAPTER 6

Interpretation and Use of the Scales for Evaluating Treatment Outcome

Once it has been determined that a child has ADHD, the next important challenge is to begin thinking of ways to bring about improvements in the child's functioning. Many different treatments are available for achieving this goal. Among these are pharmacotherapy, parent training, and classroom modifications (Barkley, 1998). In this chapter we describe how to use scores on the ADHD Rating Scale–IV to determine whether treatment has led to significant change in a child's ADHD symptoms.

Assessing the Clinical Significance of Treatment Outcome

Regardless of which treatment or combination of treatments is used, effective clinical practice dictates that some attempt be made to assess their clinical efficacy. In other words, clinicians must try to answer the question: Was treatment effective in bringing about desired changes in the child's functioning?

The manner in which this question is addressed can be highly variable. In its most basic form, clinicians can simply ask parents and teachers whether a particular treatment led to improvements in the child's home or school functioning. If the answer is "yes," the treatment worked; if "no," it did not. Obviously, this approach is highly subjective and, therefore, prone to numerous inaccuracies that can lead to faulty conclusions about treatment efficacy. A more objective approach involves the use of parent- and teacher-completed behavior rating scales, or perhaps even psychological test procedures administered to the child directly, prior to and following treatment. Although quantifying change in this way certainly increases objectivity, there remains much room for subjective clinical judgment to enter into the clinical decision-making process. For example, should any change from pretreatment to posttreatment be considered evidence of clinically significant improvement? If not, of what magnitude should the change be before one can arrive at the conclusion that treatment was successful?

Fortunately, statistical methods have been developed to assist clinicians and researchers in answering these questions. Of particular relevance for the purposes of this discussion is the Reliable Change Index (RCI) procedure for assessing clinical significance that was developed by Jacobsen and Truax (1991). According to these researchers, RCI is equal to the difference between a child's pretreatment score and posttreatment score, divided by the standard error of difference between the two test scores. When the RCI exceeds 1.96, it is unlikely that the change from pretreatment to posttreatment is due to chance ($p <$ .05). Thus, the RCI serves as a measure of the degree to which an improvement in functioning is likely due to the effects of treatment rather than to imprecise measurement.

Given its sound psychometric qualities and ease of administration, the ADHD Rating Scale–IV is especially well suited to serving as an index of treatment-induced changes in primary ADHD symptomatology. As a way of increasing its accuracy as a treatment outcome measure, we would strongly recommend using this scale in combination with the Jacobsen and Truax (1991) procedure for assessing clinical significance. To assist clinicians in making such determinations, we have calculated standard errors of difference for the Inattention, Hyperactivity–Impulsivity, and Total scores according to age and gender groupings. The standard errors of difference for the teacher version of ADHD Rating Scale–IV are presented in Table 6.1. Standard errors of difference for the parent version may be found in Table 6.2.

To calculate an RCI score for a specific child, the clinician should first subtract the pretreatment rating scale score from the posttreatment score. The resulting difference score should then be divided by the standard error of difference, as displayed in Tables 6.1 and 6.2. For example, if one were attempting to calculate an RCI for teacher ratings of a 7-year-old boy on the Inattention subscale, the standard error of difference would be 3.59 (see Table 6.1).

TABLE 6.1. Standard Errors of Difference for ADHD Rating Scale–IV Scores: School Version

Age (years)	Boys			Girls		
	IA	HI	Total	IA	HI	Total
5–7	3.59	3.85	6.53	3.41	3.56	6.08
8–10	3.99	3.95	6.93	3.42	3.01	5.64
11–13	3.80	3.30	6.05	3.17	2.74	5.11
14–18	3.41	2.98	5.43	2.47	1.67	3.55

Note. IA, Inattention score; HI, Hyperactivity–Impulsivity score.

TABLE 6.2. Standard Errors of Difference for ADHD Rating Scale–IV Scores: Home Version

Age (years)	Boys			Girls		
	IA	HI	Total	IA	HI	Total
5–7	3.37	2.94	5.46	2.96	2.39	4.47
8–10	3.54	2.77	5.37	2.88	2.01	4.12
11–13	4.16	2.93	6.19	3.39	1.84	4.29
14–18	3.55	2.29	4.91	3.03	2.02	4.24

Note. IA, Inattention score; HI, Hyperactivity–Impulsivity score.

Case Examples

To further illustrate how the ADHD Rating Scale–IV scores may be converted into RCIs and then used to assess treatment outcome, two case examples are described. The first involves the use of behavioral parent training as a treatment for home-based ADHD difficulties. In the second example, a stimulant medication trial for addressing school-based ADHD problems is discussed.

David

David is an 8-year-old third-grade boy who was referred for psychological assessment because of parent and teacher concerns about his home and school performance and behavior. The results of his initial multimethod assessment were a diagnosis of ADHD, Combined subtype, along with a secondary diagnosis of Oppositional Defiant Disorder (ODD). Together, his ADHD and ODD were making it quite difficult for his parents to control his home behavior, which in turn was contributing to their increasingly higher levels of stress. For a variety of reasons, his parents preferred not to begin a stimulant medication regimen for David. Instead, their preference was to use psychosocial treatments initially, both at home and at school. For this reason, behavioral parent training and classroom modifications were initiated. What follows is a brief description of the evaluation of his home-based treatment.

At the time of David's initial evaluation, his mother had completed the ADHD Rating Scale–IV. His Inattention score was 18, his Hyperactivity–Impulsivity score was 21, and his Total score was 39. Within 2 weeks of this evaluation, David's parents began participating in a 10-session parent training program, specifically designed for children with ADHD (Anastopoulos & Barkley, 1990). When the ninth session of this program was completed approximately 2 months later, David's mother once again rated his behavior, using the ADHD Rating Scale–IV. According to her posttreatment ratings, David's Inattention score had dropped to 14, his Hyperactivity–Impulsivity score was down to 16, and his Total score had reached 30. At face value, these changes from pretreatment to posttreatment suggested the possibility that parent training had been effective in reducing his primary ADHD symptomatology. Upon closer inspection, using RCI calculations, such conclusions seemed premature. For example, the difference in David's Inattention scores was 4. Dividing this difference by 3.54 (see Table 6.2), which is the appropriate standard error of difference for a boy his age, yielded an RCI of 1.13. Similar calculations for the pretreatment–posttreatment differences in his Hyperactivity–Impulsivity and Total scores yielded RCIs of 1.81 and 1.68. Because none of these RCIs exceeded 1.96, one could not confidently conclude that the apparent improvements in David's ADHD symptomatology were due to the effects of treatment versus those related to imprecise measurement.

Further clarification of this matter, however, occurred 1 month later when David's parents attended the 10th session of the parent training program, which was a booster session. Once again, David's mother completed the ADHD Rating Scale–IV. During this follow-up assessment, David's Inattention score was 12, his Hyperactivity–Impulsivity score was 14, and his Total score was 26. Comparisons of these scores with those observed during the initial assessment yielded RCIs of 1.69 (Inattention), 2.53 (Hyperactivity–Impulsivity), and 2.42 (Total), respectively. Thus, although there continued to be little evidence of statistically reliable change in terms of his Inattention symptoms, there was much reason to believe that the observed improvements in his Hyperactivity–Impulsivity symptoms were due to his parents' continued use and mastery of what they had learned in the parent training program.

Erika

Erika is a 10-year-old fifth-grade girl who was diagnosed with ADHD, Predominantly Inattentive subtype. Although she certainly exhibited ADHD-related problems both at home and at school, most of her difficulties occurred in the classroom setting. For this reason, Erika's parents requested that a trial of stimulant medication therapy be conducted prior to initiating any classroom modifications. A 4-week, double-blind, drug–placebo methylphenidate (Ritalin) trial was employed. During the first week of the trial she was given a low dose of stimulant medication twice a day for the entire week. In week 2 she received a placebo dose twice daily. In weeks 3 and 4 she received medium and high doses, respectively. At the end of each week, her parents and teacher completed ratings of her behavior and of possible side effects. For the purposes of this case discussion, only the teacher ratings are considered. A summary of Erika's ADHD Rating Scale–IV results, which were obtained during her initial evaluation and during the 4-week medication trial, appears in Table 6.3.

As shown in this table, Erika's Inattention score during the placebo week was only 2 points less than it had been during her initial assessment prior to the start of the medication trial. Dividing this difference by 3.42, the appropriate standard error of difference for a girl her age (see Table 6.1), yielded an RCI of .58. Similar calculations yielded placebo-week RCI scores of .33 for Hyperactivity–Impulsivity and .18 for the Total score. Thus, these changes in performance were likely due to chance fluctuations.

TABLE 6.3. Summary of ADHD Rating Scale–IV Results Obtained during Methylphenidate Trial

			Trial conditions		
	Baseline	Placebo	Low dose	Medium dose	High dose
Inattention	22	20 (.58)	21 (.29)	13 (2.63)	16 (1.75)
Hyperactivity–Impulsivity	7	8 (−.33)	6 (.33)	5 (.66)	6 (.33)
Total	29	28 (.18)	27 (.35)	18 (1.95)	22 (1.24)

Note. Reliable change scores are in parentheses.

Likewise, the RCI calculations for the low-dosage week yielded nonsignificant indices of .29 for Inattention, .33 for Hyperactivity–Impulsivity, and .35 for the Total score.

In contrast, the differences between Erika's initial scores and those obtained during the medium- and high-dosage conditions were much larger. At face value, both dosage conditions seem to have produced acceptable improvements in ADHD symptomatology. Upon closer inspection, however, important differences become evident. The RCI calculations for the medium-dosage week yielded scores of 2.63 for Inattention, .66 for Hyperactivity–Impulsivity, and 1.95 for the Total score. The corresponding RCI scores for the high dosage week were 1.75, .33, and 1.24, respectively. On the basis of these RCI calculations, therefore, it was clear that Erika's ADHD symptomatology had been significantly reduced only during the medium-dosage condition. Because somewhat fewer side effects were noted during this week as well, it was concluded that Erika would be a good candidate for a longer-term trial of methylphenidate therapy at the medium dosage level.

APPENDIX

Rating Scales
and Scoring Sheets

ADHD RATING SCALE–IV: HOME VERSION

Child's name_____ Sex: M F Age_____ Grade_____

Completed by: Mother_____ Father_____ Guardian_____ Grandparent_____

Circle the number that *best describes* your child's home behavior over the past 6 months.

	Never or rarely	Sometimes	Often	Very often
1. Fails to give close attention to details or makes careless mistakes in schoolwork.	0	1	2	3
2. Fidgets with hands or feet or squirms in seat.	0	1	2	3
3. Has difficulty sustaining attention in tasks or play activities.	0	1	2	3
4. Leaves seat in classroom or in other situations in which remaining seated is expected.	0	1	2	3
5. Does not seem to listen when spoken to directly.	0	1	2	3
6. Runs about or climbs excessively in situations in which it is inappropriate.	0	1	2	3
7. Does not follow through on instructions and fails to finish work.	0	1	2	3
8. Has difficulty playing or engaging in leisure activities quietly.	0	1	2	3
9. Has difficulty organizing tasks and activities.	0	1	2	3
10. Is "on the go" or acts as if "driven by a motor."	0	1	2	3
11. Avoids tasks (e.g., schoolwork, homework) that require sustained mental effort.	0	1	2	3
12. Talks excessively.	0	1	2	3
13. Loses things necessary for tasks or activities.	0	1	2	3
14. Blurts out answers before questions have been completed.	0	1	2	3
15. Is easily distracted.	0	1	2	3
16. Has difficulty awaiting turn.	0	1	2	3
17. Is forgetful in daily activities.	0	1	2	3
18. Interrupts or intrudes on others.	0	1	2	3

ADHD RATING SCALE–IV: HOME VERSION (Spanish)

Edad del niño/niña_____ Sexo: M F Grado____ País de origen_____

Completado por: Madre_____ Padre_____ Abuela/o_____ Otro parentesco_____

Escoja el número *que mejor describa* la conducta de su niño/niña en los últimos 6 meses.

	Nunca o rare-mente	Al-gunas veces	A menudo	Con mucha fre-cuencia
1. No logra prestar atención a detalles o es descuidado con su trabajo escolar.	0	1	2	3
2. Continuamente mueve sus manos o pies o se tuerce en el asiento.	0	1	2	3
3. Tiene dificultad en mantener su atención en las tareas o actividades de juego.	0	1	2	3
4. No permanence en su asiento en el salón de clases o en otras situaciones en las cuales se require que se mantenga sentado.	0	1	2	3
5. No parece escuchar cuando se le habla directamente.	0	1	2	3
6. Corre y se encarama en forma excesiva en situaciones en las cuales esta conducta no es apropiada.	0	1	2	3
7. No sigue instrucciones y no logra terminar su trabajo.	0	1	2	3
8. Tiene dificultad jugando o envolviéndose callá-damente en actividades recreativas o de descanso.	0	1	2	3
9. Tiene dificultad para organizar sus tareas o actividades.	0	1	2	3
10. Está siempre de prisa o actúa como si estuviera "activado por un motor."	0	1	2	3
11. Evita tareas (trabajo de la escuela) que requieren un ezfuerzo mental continuo.	0	1	2	3
12. Habla excesivamente.	0	1	2	3
13. Pierde cosas que son necesarias para sus tareas o actividades.	0	1	2	3
14. Responde impulsivamente antes de que se le termine de preguntar.	0	1	2	3
15. Se distrae fácilmente.	0	1	2	3
16. Tiene dificultad en esperar su turno.	0	1	2	3
17. Es olvidadizo con sus actividades diarias.	0	1	2	3
18. Interrumpe o se entromete sin la autorización de otros.	0	1	2	3

ADHD RATING SCALE–IV: HOME VERSION
SCORING SHEET FOR BOYS

Child's name_____ Date_____ Age_____

%ile	HI 5–7	HI 8–10	HI 11–13	HI 14–18	IA 5–7	IA 8–10	IA 11–13	IA 14–18	Total 5–7	Total 8–10	Total 11–13	Total 14–18	%ile
99+	26	25	25	19	24	26	27	25	43	49	51	41	99+
99	25	24	24	18	23	25	26	24	42	48	50	40	99
98	22	21	21	16	20	22	24	23	40	42	47	36	98
97	21	18	18	16	20	19	22	19	37	37	38	32	97
96	19	17	18	15	18	18	21	18	36	34	37	30	96
95	17	17	18	13	16	17	20	17	34	31	35	28	95
94	17	15	18	12	15	16	19	16	33	29	34	27	94
93	17	15	16	11	15	15	18	15	30	27	34	27	93
92	16	14	16	11	14	15	18	14	30	26	33	26	92
91	16	14	15	11	13	14	18	14	29	26	32	25	91
90	15	13	14	10	13	14	18	14	29	25	31	23	90
89	14	13	13	10	12	14	17	13	28	24	30	21	89
88	14	12	12	10	12	13	17	12	27	24	30	21	88
87	13	11	11	9	12	13	16	12	25	23	28	20	87
86	13	11	10	9	12	12	16	11	22	23	26	20	86
85	12	10	10	8	11	12	14	11	22	22	23	19	85
84	12	10	9	8	11	12	14	10	21	21	22	18	84
80	11	9	8	7	9	11	10	9	19	20	19	16	80
75	9	8	7	6	8	9	9	8	18	17	14	13	75
50	5	4	3	2	5	6	5	4	10	10	7	7	50
25	3	2	1	0	2	3	2	1	6	5	4	3	25
10	1	0	0	0	0	0	1	0	2	1	1	0	10
1	0	0	0	0	0	0	0	0	0	0	0	0	1

Note. HI, Hyperactivity–Impulsivity; IA, Inattention.

From *ADHD Rating Scale–IV: Checklists, Norms, and Clinical Interpretation* by George J. DuPaul, Thomas J. Power, Arthur D. Anastopoulos, and Robert Reid. Copyright 1998 by the authors. Permission to photocopy this scoring sheet is granted to purchasers of *ADHD Rating Scale–IV* for personal use only (see copyright page for details).

ADHD RATING SCALE–IV: HOME VERSION
SCORING SHEET FOR GIRLS

Child's name _____ Date _____ Age _____

%ile	HI 5–7	HI 8–10	HI 11–13	HI 14–18	IA 5–7	IA 8–10	IA 11–13	IA 14–18	Total 5–7	Total 8–10	Total 11–13	Total 14–18	%ile
99+	24	20	18	19	23	21	26	21	38	39	43	35	99+
99	23	19	17	18	22	20	25	20	37	38	42	34	99
98	20	15	12	16	18	16	21	16	30	30	28	32	98
97	17	13	11	15	16	15	19	16	29	26	24	28	97
96	14	12	11	13	15	14	17	15	29	24	23	28	96
95	14	11	10	11	14	13	16	14	28	22	22	24	95
94	13	11	9	10	13	12	15	13	27	21	21	23	94
93	13	9	9	10	12	12	13	12	24	20	20	22	93
92	12	9	8	9	11	11	12	12	23	18	19	21	92
91	11	8	8	9	11	11	11	11	21	17	19	20	91
90	11	8	8	8	10	10	11	11	20	16	18	19	90
89	10	8	7	8	10	9	11	10	19	16	18	19	89
88	9	7	7	7	9	9	10	10	19	15	17	18	88
87	9	7	6	7	9	8	10	9	19	15	17	16	87
86	9	7	6	6	9	8	10	9	19	14	16	14	86
85	9	7	6	6	8	8	10	9	18	14	16	14	85
84	9	6	6	6	8	8	9	8	17	14	15	13	84
80	8	6	5	5	7	7	8	7	15	12	13	12	80
75	7	5	4	5	6	6	7	6	13	11	11	10	75
50	4	2	2	2	3	3	3	3	7	6	5	5	50
25	2	1	0	0	1	1	1	1	4	2	2	2	25
10	0	0	0	0	0	0	0	0	1	0	0	0	10
1	0	0	0	0	0	0	0	0	0	0	0	0	1

Note. HI, Hyperactivity–Impulsivity; IA, Inattention.

ADHD RATING SCALE–IV: SCHOOL VERSION

Child's name_____ Sex: M F Age_____ Grade_____

Completed by: _____

Circle the number that *best describes* this student's school behavior over the past 6 months (or since the beginning of the school year).

	Never or rarely	Sometimes	Often	Very often
1. Fails to give close attention to details or makes careless mistakes in schoolwork.	0	1	2	3
2. Fidgets with hands or feet or squirms in seat.	0	1	2	3
3. Has difficulty sustaining attention in tasks or play activities.	0	1	2	3
4. Leaves seat in classroom or in other situations in which remaining seated is expected.	0	1	2	3
5. Does not seem to listen when spoken to directly.	0	1	2	3
6. Runs about or climbs excessively in situations in which it is inappropriate.	0	1	2	3
7. Does not follow through on instructions and fails to finish work.	0	1	2	3
8. Has difficulty playing or engaging in leisure activities quietly.	0	1	2	3
9. Has difficulty organizing tasks and activities.	0	1	2	3
10. Is "on the go" or acts as if "driven by a motor."	0	1	2	3
11. Avoids tasks (e.g., schoolwork, homework) that require sustained mental effort.	0	1	2	3
12. Talks excessively.	0	1	2	3
13. Loses things necessary for tasks or activities.	0	1	2	3
14. Blurts out answers before questions have been completed.	0	1	2	3
15. Is easily distracted.	0	1	2	3
16. Has difficulty awaiting turn.	0	1	2	3
17. Is forgetful in daily activities.	0	1	2	3
18. Interrupts or intrudes on others.	0	1	2	3

ADHD RATING SCALE–IV: SCHOOL VERSION
SCORING SHEET FOR BOYS

Child's name_____ Date_____ Age_____

%ile	HI 5–7	HI 8–10	HI 11–13	HI 14–18	IA 5–7	IA 8–10	IA 11–13	IA 14–18	Total 5–7	Total 8–10	Total 11–13	Total 14–18	%ile
99+	27	27	27	25	27	27	27	27	52	54	54	52	99+
99	27	27	27	25	27	27	27	27	51	53	53	51	99
98	27	27	25	21	26	27	27	27	51	53	49	44	98
97	27	26	23	21	24	26	27	25	50	51	44	43	97
96	25	26	21	21	24	26	25	24	48	50	42	39	96
95	24	26	20	20	23	25	25	23	46	50	40	39	95
94	23	25	18	19	23	25	24	22	44	48	39	35	94
93	22	25	18	17	22	25	24	21	41	46	38	34	93
92	21	24	18	16	22	24	23	21	40	45	37	33	92
91	21	23	17	14	21	24	23	20	40	45	36	32	91
90	20	22	17	13	21	24	23	20	39	44	36	31	90
89	20	21	16	12	20	24	22	19	38	42	34	30	89
88	19	21	16	12	20	24	21	18	38	41	33	29	88
87	18	20	16	12	19	23	20	18	37	41	33	28	87
86	18	19	15	11	18	22	20	18	37	40	32	28	86
85	17	19	14	10	18	22	19	17	35	39	32	27	85
84	17	18	14	10	17	21	19	17	34	38	31	26	84
80	16	16	12	8	16	19	17	15	30	34	28	23	80
75	14	13	10	7	15	17	16	12	28	30	25	20	75
50	6	5	3	1	7	9	8	7	13	15	12	9	50
25	1	2	1	0	2	2	2	2	4	5	3	2	25
10	0	0	0	0	0	0	0	0	0	1	0	0	10
1	0	0	0	0	0	0	0	0	0	0	0	0	1

Note. HI, Hyperactivity–Impulsivity; IA, Inattention.

From *ADHD Rating Scale–IV: Checklists, Norms, and Clinical Interpretation* by George J. DuPaul, Thomas J. Power, Arthur D. Anastopoulos, and Robert Reid. Copyright 1998 by the authors. Permission to photocopy this scoring sheet is granted to purchasers of *ADHD Rating Scale–IV* for personal use only (see copyright page for details).

ADHD RATING SCALE–IV: SCHOOL VERSION
SCORING SHEET FOR GIRLS

Child's name_____ Date_____ Age_____

%ile	HI 5–7	HI 8–10	HI 11–13	HI 14–18	IA 5–7	IA 8–10	IA 11–13	IA 14–18	Total 5–7	Total 8–10	Total 11–13	Total 14–18	%ile
99+	27	27	26	16	26	27	27	22	49	52	50	34	99+
99	26	27	25	15	25	27	27	21	48	51	49	33	99
98	26	25	24	13	24	26	24	18	47	50	42	28	98
97	25	25	22	11	23	25	23	18	45	48	41	27	97
96	25	22	20	11	23	25	22	17	44	44	40	26	96
95	23	20	17	10	21	24	21	16	44	38	39	25	95
94	22	18	17	9	21	22	20	16	41	36	35	22	94
93	21	17	15	9	21	21	19	15	40	35	31	22	93
92	21	14	12	9	20	20	18	14	38	33	30	20	92
91	20	12	12	8	20	20	18	13	37	32	30	20	91
90	19	12	11	8	19	19	17	13	36	30	27	18	90
89	18	12	10	8	19	18	17	12	35	29	25	18	89
88	16	10	10	5	17	16	16	11	33	28	23	17	88
87	15	10	9	5	17	15	15	11	32	26	22	17	87
86	14	9	8	5	16	14	15	10	31	25	21	16	86
85	13	9	8	4	16	14	14	10	29	20	21	14	85
84	13	8	7	4	16	13	13	10	28	20	21	14	84
80	11	6	6	3	13	10	11	8	23	16	17	11	80
75	9	5	5	2	11	9	9	7	20	14	14	9	75
50	2	1	1	0	4	3	4	2	7	4	5	3	50
25	0	0	0	0	0	0	1	0	2	1	1	0	25
10	0	0	0	0	0	0	0	0	0	0	0	0	10
1	0	0	0	0	0	0	0	0	0	0	0	0	1

Note. HI, Hyperactivity–Impulsivity; IA, Inattention.

From *ADHD Rating Scale-IV: Checklists, Norms, and Clinical Interpretation* by George J. DuPaul, Thomas J. Power, Arthur D. Anastopoulos, and Robert Reid. Copyright 1998 by the authors. Permission to photocopy this scoring sheet is granted to purchasers of *ADHD Rating Scale-IV* for personal use only (see copyright page for details).

References

Achenbach, T. M. (1991a). *Integrative guide for the 1991 CBCL/4-18, YSR, and TRF Profiles.* Burlington: University of Vermont, Department of Psychiatry.

Achenbach, T. M. (1991b). *Manual for the Child Behavior Checklist/4-18 and 1991 Profile.* Burlington: University of Vermont, Department of Psychiatry.

Achenbach, T. M. (1991c). *Manual for the Teacher's Report Form and 1991 Profile.* Burlington: University of Vermont, Department of Psychiatry.

American Psychiatric Association. (1968). *Diagnostic and statistical manual of mental disorders* (2nd ed.). Washington, DC: Author.

American Psychiatric Association. (1980). *Diagnostic and statistical manual of mental disorders* (3rd ed.). Washington, DC: Author.

American Psychiatric Association. (1987). *Diagnostic and statistical manual of mental disorders* (3rd ed., rev.). Washington, DC: Author.

American Psychiatric Association. (1994). *Diagnostic and statistical manual of mental disorders* (4th ed.). Washington, DC: Author.

Anastopoulos, A. D., & Barkley, R. A. (1990). Counseling and training parents. In R. A. Barkley, *Attention-deficit hyperactivity disorder: A handbook for diagnosis and treatment* (pp. 397–431). New York: Guilford Press.

Barkley, R. A. (1990). *Attention-deficit hyperactivity disorder: A handbook for diagnosis and treatment.* New York: Guilford Press.

Barkley, R. A. (1997). Behavioral inhibition, sustained attention, and executive functions: Constructing a unifying theory of ADHD. *Psychological Bulletin, 121,* 65–94.

Barkley, R. A. (1998). *Attention-deficit hyperactivity disorder: A handbook for diagnosis and treatment* (2nd ed.). New York: Guilford Press.

Bauermeister, J. J., Bird, H. R., Canino, G., Rubio-Stipec, M., Bravo, M., & Alegria, M. (1995). Dimensions of attention deficit hyperactivity disorder: Findings from teacher and parent reports in a community sample. *Journal of Clinical Child Psychology, 24,* 264–271.

Baumgaertel, A., Wolraich, M. L., & Dietrich, M. (1995). Comparison of diagnostic criteria for attention deficit disorders in a German elementary school sample. *Journal of the American Academy of Child and Adolescent Psychiatry, 34,* 629–638.

Bollen, K. A. (1990). Overall fit in covariance structure models: Two types of sample size effects. *Psychological Bulletin, 107,* 256–259.

Brito, G. N. O., Pinto, R. C. A., & Lins, M. F. C. (1995). A behavioral assessment scale of attention deficit disorder in Brazilian children based on DSM-III-R criteria. *Journal of Abnormal Child Psychology, 23,* 509–521.

Browne, M. W., & Cudeck, R. (1993). Alternative ways of assessing model fit. In K. A. Bollen & J. S. Long (Eds.), *Testing stucture equation models* (pp. 136–162). London: Sage.

Chen, W. J., Faraone, S. V., Biederman, J., & Tsuang, M. T. (1994). Diagnostic accuracy of the Child Behavior Checklist Scales for attention-deficit hyperactivity disorder: A receiver operating characteristic analysis. *Journal of Consulting and Clinical Psychology, 62,* 1017–1025.

Conners, C. K. (1989). *Conners Rating Scales manual.* North Tonawanda, NY: Multi-Health Systems.

DuPaul, G. J. (1991). Parent and teacher ratings of ADHD symptoms: Psychometric properties in a community-based sample. *Journal of Clinical Child Psychology, 20,* 245–253.

DuPaul, G. J., Anastopoulos, A. D., Power, T. J., Reid, R., Ikeda, M., & McGoey, K. (1998). Parent ratings of attention-deficit/hyperactivity disorder symptoms: Factor structure and normative data. *Journal of Psychopathology and Behavioral Assessment, 20,* 83–102.

DuPaul, G. J., Power, T. J., Anastopoulos, A. D., Reid, R., McGoey, K., & Ikeda, M. (1997). Teacher ratings of attention-deficit/hyperactivity disorder: Factor structure and normative data. *Psychological Assessment, 9,* 436–444.

DuPaul, G. J., Power, T. J., McGoey, K., Ikeda, M., & Anastopoulos, A. D. (1998). Reliability and validity of parent and teacher ratings of attention-deficit/hyperactivity disorder symptoms. *Journal of Psychoeducational Assessment, 16,* 55–68.

DuPaul, G. J., & Stoner, G. (1994). *ADHD in the schools: Assessment and intervention strategies.* New York: Guilford Press.

Eiraldi, R. B., Power, T. J., & Nezu, C. M. (1997). Patterns of comorbidity associated with subtypes of attention-deficit/hyperactivity disorder among 6–12-year-old children. *Journal of the American Academy of Child and Adolescent Psychiatry, 36,* 503–514.

Frick, P. J., Lahey, B. B., Applegate, B., Kerdyck, L., Ollendick, T., Hynd, G. W., Garfinkel, B., Greenhill, L., Biederman, J., Barkley, R. A., McBurnett, K., Newcorn, J., & Waldman, I. (1994). DSM-IV field trials for the disruptive behavior disorders: Symptom utility estimates. *Journal of the American Academy of Child and Adolescent Psychiatry, 33,* 529–539.

Gaub, M., & Carlson, C. L. (1997). Behavioral characteristics of DSM-IV ADHD subtypes in a school-based population. *Journal of Abnormal Child Psychology, 25,* 103–112.

Gorsuch, R. (1983). *Factor analysis.* Hillsdale, NJ: Erlbaum.

Hinshaw, S. P. (1994). *Attention deficits and hyperactivity in children.* Thousand Oaks, CA: Sage.

Hollingshead, A. B. (1975). *Four factor index of social status.* New Haven, CT: Yale University Press.

Jacobsen, N. S., & Truax, P. (1991). Clinical significance: A statistical approach to defining meaningful change in psychotherapy research. *Journal of Consulting and Clinical Psychology, 59,* 12–19.

Joreskog, K., & Sorbom, D. (1993). *LISREL 8.* Hillsdale, NJ: Erlbaum.

Kaufman, A. S., & Kaufman, N. L. (1990). *Kaufman Brief Intelligence Test.* Circle Pines, MN: American Guidance Service.

Lahey, B. B., Applegate, B., McBurnett, K., Biederman, J., Greenhill, L., Hynd, G. W., Barkley, R. A., Newcorn, J., Jensen, P., Richters, J., Garfinkel, B., Kerdyk, L., Frick, P. J., Ollendick, T., Perez, D., Hart, E. L., Waldman, I., & Schaffer, D. (1994). DSM-IV field trials for attention-deficit hyperactivity disorder in children and adolescents. *American Journal of Psychiatry, 151,* 1673–1685.

Lahey, B. B., Pelham, W. E., Schaughency, E. A., Atkins, M. S., Murphy, H. A., Hynd, G. W., Russo, M., Hartdagen, S., & Lorys-Vernon, A. (1988). Dimensions and types of attention deficit disorder. *Journal of the American Academy of Child and Adolescent Psychiatry, 27,* 330–335.

Laurent, J., Landau, S., & Stark, K. D. (1993). Conditional probabilities in the diagnosis of depressive and anxiety disorders in children. *School Psychology Review, 22,* 98–114.

Marsh, H. W., Balla, J. R., & McDonald, R. P. (1988). Goodness-of-fit indexes in confirmatory factor analysis: The effect of sample size. *Psychological Bulletin, 103,* 391–410.

McCarney, S. B. (1989). *Attention Deficit Disorder Evaluation Scale (ADDES).* Columbia, MO: Hawthorne Educational Services.

Power, T. J., Andrews, T. J., Eiraldi, R. B., Doherty, B. J., Ikeda, M. J., DuPaul, G. J., & Landau, S. (in press). Evaluating ADHD using multiple informants: The incremental utility of combining teacher with parent reports. *Psychological Assessment.*

Power, T. J., Doherty, B. J., Panichelli-Mindel, S. M., Karustis, J. L., Eiraldi, R. B., Anastopoulos, A. D., & DuPaul, G. J. (1998). Integrating parent and teacher reports in the diagnostic assessment of ADHD. *Journal of Psychopathology and Behavioral Assessment, 20,* 57–81.

Rapport, M. D., DuPaul, G. J., & Kelly, K. L. (1989). Attention-Deficit Hyperactivity Disorder and methylphenidate: The relationship between gross body weight and drug response in children. *Psychopharmacology Bulletin, 25,* 285–290.

Raykov, T., & Widaman, K. F. (1995). Issues in applied structural equation modeling research. *Structural Equation Modeling, 2,* 289–318.

Reich, W., Shayka, M. A., & Taibleson, C. (1991). *Diagnostic Interview for Children and Adolescents–DSM-III-R Version (Parent Form).* St. Louis, MO: Washington University Division of Child Psychiatry.

Reid, R. (1995). Assessment of ADHD with culturally different groups: The use of behavior rating scales. *School Psychology Review, 24,* 537–560.

Reid, R., DuPaul, G. J., Power, T. J., Anastopoulos, A. D., Rodgers-Adkinson, D., Noll, M. B., & Riccio, C. (1998). Assessing culturally different students for Attention-Deficit/Hyperactivity Disorder using behavior rating scales. *Journal of Abnormal Child Psychology, 26,* 187–198.

Shaywitz, S. E., Shaywitz, B. A., Schnell, C., & Towle, V. R. (1988). Concurrent and predictive validity of the Yale Children's Inventory: An instrument to assess children with attentional deficits and learning disabilities. *Pediatrics, 81,* 562–571.

Taylor, E., & Sandberg, S. (1984). Hyperactive behavior in English schoolchildren: A questionnaire survey. *Journal of Abnormal Child Psychology, 12,* 143–156.

Ullmann, R. K., Sleator, E. K., & Sprague, R. L. (1991). *ADD-H Comprehensive Teacher's Rating Scale–ACTeRS.* Champaign, IL: MetriTech.

Verhulst, F. C., & Koot, H. M. (1992). *Child psychiatric epidemiology: Concepts, methods, and findings.* Newbury Park, CA: Sage.

Wolraich, M. L., Hannah, J. N., Pinnock, T. Y., Baumgaertel, A., & Brown, J. (1996). Comparison of diagnostic criteria for attention-deficit hyperactivity disorder in a county-wide sample. *Journal of the American Academy of Child and Adolescent Psychiatry, 35,* 319–324.

About the Authors

GEORGE J. DUPAUL, PHD, is a professor of school psychology and coordinator of the School Psychology Program at Lehigh University in Bethlehem, PA. He is author or coauthor of numerous publications related to the assessment and treatment of ADHD, including *ADHD in the Schools: Assessment and Intervention Strategies* and the instructional videos *Assessing ADHD in the Schools* and *Classroom Interventions for ADHD.*

THOMAS J. POWER, PHD, is codirector of the ADHD/School Problems Program and acting director of the Section of Pediatric Psychology at Children's Seashore House of the Children's Hospital of Philadelphia, PA. Faculty appointments include assistant professor of school psychology in pediatrics at the University of Pennsylvania School of Medicine and adjunct associate professor of school psychology at Lehigh University. Dr. Power is currently associate editor of *School Psychology Review* and has authored numerous publications related to the assessment and treatment of ADHD.

ARTHUR D. ANASTOPOULOS, PHD, is an associate professor in the Department of Psychology at the University of North Carolina at Greensboro, where he also directs an ADHD specialty clinic for children, adolescents, and adults. An active researcher, Dr. Anastopoulos has given numerous presentations at scientific meetings and has authored more than 35 journal articles and book chapters on the topic of ADHD. He is the first author of a forthcoming text entitled *Assessing Attention-Deficit/Hyperactivity Disorder.*

ROBERT REID, PHD, is an associate professor in the Department of Special Education and Communication Disorders at the University of Nebraska—Lincoln. His interests center on treatment of attention-related problems and cognitive strategy instruction.